JUGGLING WISDOM

By

Andrew Giordano

Keep being awesome!

Andrew

Published by Youth Circus Project
Made in Canada.
2021

Copyright © 2021 by ANDREW GIORDANO

Cover Artist: Amanda Worr
Illustrations: Ely Sea

ISBN: 978-1-7778083-2-7

YOUTH CIRCUS PROJECT

Email: JugglingAndrew@gmail.com

Printed by IngramSpark

Contents

PRELUDE 3

INTRODUCTION 7

PART ONE: BELIEVE IT'S POSSIBLE 21

PART TWO: DROP THE BALL 53

PART THREE: CELEBRATE! 93

CONCLUSION 128

AFTERWORD 135

APPENDIX 139

To my younger self, who had the grit and the inclination to get out there and find a better answer.

Prelude

"Do it!"
"Come on man, what are you waiting for?"
"Hey, is he gonna do it or what?"

    I'm starting to lose the crowd, who are already hyped up like crazy. They're a pretty demanding audience. The kind that it's impossible to please - no matter what I do, they only seem to want more. The sweat is rolling down my face, dripping into my eyes and down off my chin. My heart is pounding intensely. The wind is very strong. I'm 17 stories above the ground, on the rooftop lounge of an upscale hotel in downtown Toronto...
    I've been hired to demonstrate a newly released product line - a series of accessories for iphones that allow you to strap your phone to your chest so you can take selfies while snowboarding or whatever the heck else. In this case, I'm demoing the device by strapping a phone to my chest and taking a video of me balancing on a one-inch slackline approximately 200 feet above the ground, while I juggle razor-sharp knives in front of a live audience. I have literally never done this before. The first time I do it will be right here, right now.
    To make matters worse, someone else set up my slackline, and it wasn't calibrated even close to how I usually do it. I'm way out of my league here, and genuinely unsure how I'm going to pull this off. As I'm sure you can imagine, my anxiety level is absolutely through the roof.

Cut scene

> *I'm in the checkout line at Food Basics, and it's a busy day. I have about a million and a half groceries in my cart. There's a long line of customers behind me. They also have full carts, and I can tell that they're anxious to get their shopping done and get out of there. As I'm unloading my cart onto the conveyor belt, I can feel all the eyes on me. Everyone is watching and judging me, not only on my groceries, but on how I lay them out on the belt. I can feel it. I don't even need to look up to know that everybody there is frustrated and exasperated by my existence, and the fact that I'm holding them up. I almost feel like loading my groceries back into my cart and wheeling it to the back of the line, just so that I don't have to feel this anxiety. But that's no good - by the time I get to the front, there will just be a new set of people that I'm holding up. I want to crawl under a rock and never be seen again. Again, my anxiety level is through the roof.*

Believe it or not, both of these stories are examples of typical anxiety experiences of mine. The difference between the first and the second stories is only a few years. The grocery story was taken before my journey began, while the insanely dangerous rooftop slackline knife juggling was taken from the middle of my journey. Both are true. And it's also true that both were fully terrifying to me. Gonna-have-a-heartattack-I'm-so-anxious level of terrifying. Maybe you can identify with my grocery line story. Maybe you can identify with both stories. Maybe your trigger isn't the grocery line or juggling knives where nobody has any business juggling knives. Maybe it's having to go to school. Or work. Maybe it's your parents, your teachers, your friends, your boss, your coworkers. Maybe it's yourself.

Or maybe you don't have anxiety at all. But if you're that lucky, I can pretty well guarantee that someone you know very well struggles with it. It's estimated that one in five people struggle with an anxiety disorder. Honestly, I think that's a pretty low estimate. As I'm finishing writing this book, it's nearly a year into the Covid-19 pandemic. As if people didn't already have enough to worry about, now we've also got the very real possibility of death, total isolation, loss of work, loss of purpose. Suicide rates and drug use have risen, as well as domestic violence and who knows what else. It's clear that, if we don't find a better way to relate to our anxiety, we're going to continue to slowly implode, both on an individual and on a collective scale.

If you have a mind, this book is for you. If you experience anxiety, I propose a framework that can help you to take your power back. If you don't, I hope that this book gives you a window into, and a sense of compassion for those around you who do.

To be clear, I am not promising to eliminate anxiety. Anxiety doesn't work that way. What I *am* proposing to do is to help shift *which kinds of situations cause anxiety*. To give you some breathing room so you can feel that living a happy and fulfilled life is possible. Anxiety is a bit like a strong wind - if you let it, it will push you around until you end up hiding behind some kind of shelter. That shelter could be anything - alcohol, drugs, video games, Netflix, even relationships. And it's all too easy to get stuck there - those things are comforting, predictable, and really *do* take your mind off the storm. There's nothing wrong with any of those things. But if you don't make a plan, you may find yourself so afraid of the wind that you never feel like you *can* leave your shelter(s) of choice. And the longer you stay there, the harder it gets. Trust me.

To keep with my analogy, you can't control the wind, or take the wind away. It'll always be there. But you *can* develop tactics to get to places that are more fulfilling, and much less windy in general. The only difficulty is that you're going to have to venture out into the cold harsh wind to get to those places. The good news is that the wind itself has no power to harm you. It is just a feeling, and no matter how bad it feels, it always changes over time.

Juggling Wisdom is no panacea - it's not a quick fix, nor is it easy. Practicing these principles, you will come up against yourself over and over again. It'll hurt. It'll suck. You'll feel like a fool. You'll be self-conscious and doubt whether this is worth all the hassle. But, if I've done my job well enough, you'll have fun along the way. You'll absolutely learn more about yourself and what you're *really* capable of (as opposed to the limits your anxiety puts on you). The process is designed to be fun and worthwhile in itself, independent of the results you'll experience. If you can hold these words in a spirit of lightness and play, I promise it'll be a lot easier than if you make it heavy.

At this point in my career, I have shared Juggling Wisdom with tens (maybe hundreds) of thousands of bodies. Often the results are instantaneous - people catch themselves making "can't" statements, and immediately prove themselves wrong by doing something super-impressive that they never knew they could do. They find themselves smiling and laughing and being cheered on by their peers. Sometimes the experience is life-changing.

If you truly practice Juggling Wisdom, I believe that your horizons of possibility will expand tremendously. I believe that limitations that you thought were absolute will drop away like imagined things. If you take these principles to heart and practice them consistently over time, I believe that the situations that currently cause anxiety for you will become a whole heck of a lot easier, and your new challenges will be lightyears ahead of where you ever thought you'd be.

Now, you may be wondering how my teaser story ends. The one about juggling the knives 200 feet in the air, not the grocery one. Well, I'm afraid that there's a whole lot of context I need to explain before you can appreciate the ending. Read on, and I promise you'll be rewarded!

Introduction

Hello there! My name is Andrew and I'm a professional circus artist. Not the greatest you'll ever see, but I've definitely got a few tricks worth watching. When I perform, my stage name is Andrew the Absolutely Normal. It's a joke that nobody ever gets – which probably makes it a bad joke. But I'm not willing to give it up. Why? Because I'm trying to make a point. The point I'm trying so unsuccessfully to make is about the reaction that I often hear from my audiences. When I juggle any more than three balls (I occasionally juggle up to 7 in performance), or if I'm incorporating "danger" by juggling knives or flaming torches on my 6-foot unicycle, people almost inevitably pull out the "t word" on me. Not Terrific, Terrifying, or even Terrible (funny how these are all incarnations of the same word). No, they call me "talented", and I hate it. I hate it to death, because it's an incorrect, and frankly, insulting assumption. It's a dismissal of the **thousands** of hours that I had to put in. My ability to juggle, ride a unicycle, or perform acrobatics didn't come from being born with some strange characteristic. It came from a whole lot of fumbling around until I unknowingly followed some secret recipe, which I've taken the time to record and explain in this book.

I won't deny that people have propensities for different activities, in that they learn more quickly and seem better suited to them. For example, some people have a propensity for contorting their bodies into weird shapes for entertainment. Personally, I don't relish the thought of fitting my entire body into a cheerios box. Needless to say, I don't have a propensity for contortion. Nor do I have a propensity for juggling. I am neither quicker nor better suited to juggle, except insofar as I have a healthy body with functional arms, eyes, and brain (though this last point is questionable on some days... more on that later.) In fact, it has taken me several times as long to learn most tricks as the people around me. I measured at one point and concluded that I learn juggling skills at roughly a quarter the speed of your average juggler.

I know that my audience means well when they say this, but I still feel insulted. So much so that I rarely perform any more. This may seem an overreaction, but in order to understand it, you need to understand why I took up juggling in the first place. So here's a brief version of my story:

The Spark

I'm in my first year of university, studying psychology, and my life feels like it's in grey. There is no colour yet, only the hope of finding something important enough to me that it might introduce the sense of life that I seem to see in those around me. Fortunately for me, I don't have to wait long – I find it in my second month, in the most unexpected place. My parents have bought tickets for the family to see Cirque Du Soleil's "Corteo". I had always known of Cirque du Soleil, and had caught glimpses of their shows on TV as a child, following which I have vague memories of trying unsuccessfully to pull off a handstand, only to crash into the furniture and be scolded by my mother. Needless to say, I was looking forward to it. However, I realize in the moment that I step into the tent that nothing has prepared me for this experience.

The atmosphere is alive with energy. The circular stage with runway divides the tent and the audience into two sections. Masking the circus ring are two beautiful translucent curtains depicting an enormous renaissance painting complete with angels and cherubs. The story of this show is a clown dreaming of his own funeral. Clowns roam through the audience, mourning excessively, squirting their "tears" into the audience via concealed tubes in their sleeves. Immediately, my eyes are peeled and all senses are fully online. Mournful organ music resonates in the background as we take our seats.

The curtains lift and the show begins. Acrobats, jugglers, dancers, and clowns march across the smoke-filled stage. Three beautiful chandeliers hang low, casting the scene with dim light. On their way past, three beautiful dancers each grab hold of a chandelier, taking it with them. Then, they raise into the air as my stomach leaps. What follows is a gorgeous and graceful aerial dance featuring swinging chandeliers with real live people hanging upside-down, turning and holding with one hand while they sail through the air, at times overtop the audience.

Act after act fills me with wonder – I had never truly seen such feats before. My scattered glimpses on the TV were nothing compared to seeing these live artists right in front of my face, doing the impossible. At the time, I had no words to describe it. These people were performing impossible feats stacked on top of impossible feats until it felt as if this must not be the real world. I learned later that this is the definition of **awe***. It was ineffable and almost incomprehensible. It shattered all my ideas of what's possible and what's impossible. In those moments, I became a child again, the world filled with wonder and magic.*

Near the end of the show, I thought I had seen it all – what could possibly top the 4 jugglers who kept 20 objects in the air together? Or the highwire act? Or actual triple backflips performed on a teeter-totter? But what followed was the most spectacular thing I'd seen in my life – a free-standing ladder act. You know those A-frame ladders? It wasn't one of those. It was one half of an A-frame. And you know how those are usually leaning against something? Yeah, that wasn't it either. It was just him and his ladder on the stage. He starts climbing the ladder step by step, wiggling it back and forth to balance. He manages to climb all the way up one side and backwards down the other. I can't believe that this is happening, and that I get to see it. His next trick has him climbing all the way up the ladder and slipping his body, bent backwards, between the top and second-from-top rungs. Balancing in a terribly dangerous back arch that would be fatal if he fell, he readies himself. Jumping, he pulls himself in a backflip over the top rung to land on the other side without falling. My jaw drops. He moves on to do a full handstand on the very top of the ladder. My stomach drops. For his finale, he discards his 8-foot ladder and moves on to a 15-foot ladder. There are no nets, no mats, and no safety wires. Surely this must be a joke – how could anyone do this?! Rung by rung, one precarious step at a time, he climbs all the way up, where he places his feet on the tiny platforms at the very top. He seems to be walking on the clouds, effortlessly, his face filled with joy.

Leaving the show that night, I was transformed. I had no way of knowing the incredible journey and wild experiences that would result from this show, but I finally had my first sense of colour. When I returned home, the whole world was suffused with possibility. Doors were open that had never been open before. I finally had something that seemed unquestionably worth doing. I dug up my old juggling balls and re-learned how to juggle 3 (I had learned in elementary school from a guest speaker). I bought a unicycle and taught myself how to ride it. Armed with new knowledge from online videos, I spent terrifying hours in public parks, teaching myself how to do a backflip. I taught myself how to hold a handstand, increased my juggling patterns from 3 balls to 4, to 5, 6, 7, and eventually 8.

Each step of the way I was astounded by what was possible. Each time I achieved a new feat, I was tempted to think that I had reached the pinnacle of my capacity. But around each corner was the thrilling possibility of the next feat. If I can juggle and ride a unicycle, could I possibly do both at the same time? If I can ride a small unicycle, can I ride a 6-foot tall one? If I can juggle balls, can I also juggle rings, clubs, knives, flaming torches? The answer to each turned out to be: with practice, yes! (As an aside, at the time of writing this book, I've just set 5 world records for juggling on a tall unicycle!)

Eventually I had to come to terms with this obsession. Was this just a fun experiment? What was my end goal? Here comes the second piece of the puzzle: studying psychology, now in my second year, I'm reading my textbook for Abnormal Psychology, when my jaw drops. As I read the section on anxiety disorders, specifically social anxiety disorder, I have a shocking experience that I'm reading about myself in the third person. Word for word, it's as if the authors have somehow reached into my head and are telling me what my own experience in the world is, in more eloquent terms than I'd even been able to describe it.

Wow, so I have a social anxiety disorder... That explains a lot. See, I'd always been told I was shy, I thought that's what the term meant – that the extreme anxiety and panic that come when I'm around people is just what happens when one is "shy". The authors write that one of the most frustrating aspects of this condition is that, even **knowing** that one has this condition, even **knowing** that it is irrational, the symptoms persist. It is not something that one can "think" their way out of.

Now I have a decision to make: knowing this about myself, do I continue on my path of pursuing circus arts? Or do I choose a more "realistic" option? Taking stock of my life, I realized that I spent far more time juggling, unicycling, and acrobat-ing than I did in class. But how could I ever become a performer when I regularly experience panic attacks and need to escape social situations? I had a few incidents of taking the bus to school, and having to get off after only one stop because I couldn't cope with the anxiety and panic that I felt just by being around people. Without performing. I couldn't do parties, social events, or bar nights without panicking and having to leave. So how the heck could I possibly make this work?

You already know how this story ends, but I didn't. I was tortured and torn apart at the thought of putting myself through so much hardship to follow this path. But even stronger than that was my conviction that I'd finally found something worth doing. That I couldn't give up on this thing that meant so much to me, no matter what the cost. So I pushed through the difficulty and took some steps. I started practicing in public more often, until it became natural. I made some friends who were interested in learning with me, and was able to make my practice more social.

My first circus performance was for the half-time of a university basketball game. I legitimately thought I was going to have a heart-attack, I was so nervous. But I committed. And I did it. And when the show was over, it was one of the greatest victories I'd ever achieved in my life. My heart was pounding so hard that I thought that I would die. But at the end of the show, I was still standing. In fact, I was exhilarated! It was both

> *the biggest relief and the biggest sense of exhilaration that I had ever experienced.*

I decided that this was my purpose in life: to spread the message that we are all capable of so much more than we think. And that achieving these things doesn't have to be work: it can be fun, playful, a celebration. That is what circus means to me. In the years that followed, I have travelled the world and performed for countless audiences. I have also had the honour and the privilege of sharing a message that is uplifting and empowering to listeners of all genders, skin colours, ability levels, ages, and body types.

My quest is to share principles that are universally true and empowering, which help to drive us both as individuals and as a collective, toward more rich and fulfilling lives. It is my hope that the principles I share in this book will help you to discover a world of untapped richness and possibility in your own life.

Why Juggling?

Let's face it: personal development can seem heavy, can't it? For a lot of people, this field carries with it a whole lot of baggage, assumptions, and overall unpleasantness. Diets that don't work, resolutions that fail, and strategies that propel us toward the mysterious and elusive idea of "success", in my experience, have created an atmosphere of cynicism around self improvement. Even the idea of personal development suggests a deficit, doesn't it? There's a hidden (and sometimes not-so-hidden) suggestion that, without the latest fad, tip, or trick, our lives are shamefully deficient.

One of the things that I've found to be universally true is that humans are automatically inclined toward growth, learning and development, *unless something happens to get in the way*. I think that, most often, the *something* that gets in the way is shame. Hell, our whole culture runs on shame! Looking back through the ages of the personal development industry, there are too many examples of messages that have shame at their core: You are not good enough… unless you buy my book, try my diet, my fix, my cure. And there's a huge cost to this: if my infallible cure doesn't work on you, there must be something uniquely wrong with *you*. And you may just walk away from the experiment feeling defeated, and like you shouldn't have bothered in the first place. Now you're left in your "norm of deficiency", without any hope for anything better.

When we internalize these messages, of course it turns us off from trying! Sitting in our state of deficiency may be painful, but trying to fix it and failing is even **more** painful. Growth, it seems, must be for other people. Healthy and fit bodies must just be something that other people have.

Juggling is my way of trying to remind us all that growth and development doesn't have to be so heavy. That you don't have to start from a place of deficiency.

My work with children over the years has led me to the observation that they are particularly good at learning, and pick up so many things more quickly than adults. I believe there are two reasons behind this:

• Children don't carry with them the same baggage that we, as adults carry. Their minds aren't so full of impossibilities, dead ends, or insurmountable barriers.

• Children learn by playing. "Mistakes" carry no cost with them. There is no sense of shame or defeat attached to trying something that doesn't work. If their blocks don't stack up the way they tried, they either try again or cheerfully move on to the next experiment.

I believe very strongly that, in order to achieve the best results, we need to lower the cost of our "failure" and increase the rewards of our "success". I put these in quotations because it's worth getting clear on our definitions, which we'll get to next. Juggling is a return to our first (and most fun) mode of learning: play. When we break down all of the heaviness involved in learning, it becomes more accessible and more rewarding to more people, and that makes it more universal. And I believe that the fruits of this learning are spectacular and worthy of celebration.

The Importance of Definitions

I heard once that thought is determined by language. That the shape and connections of the things in our heads are bound to the words we use to describe them. I've never been sure if that is wholly correct, but it certainly seems to have enough truth that it's worth talking about. Your concept of the word "juggle" provides the foundation of your assessment of whether you can do it or not. If you think I mean you need to do something really difficult, you're going to hold it in a different place in your mind than if you think I'm talking about throwing a single ball in interesting ways.

I've noticed that the biggest objection people have when I suggest that they can juggle is their incorrect assumption that "juggling" means throwing and catching 3 balls in a very specific pattern, known as the "cascade". That's like defining "music" as opera only and dismissing every other variety of music. Both are ridiculous. I want to take some time to clear things up so that we're not thinking of totally different things when I say "juggling".

I don't purport to have the best or most accurate definition of the word "juggle", but I have one that has served me and my students very well over the years of my teaching. In fact, let me introduce it through a quick story about my first breakthrough in teaching juggling.

Mistaken Goals

I was frustrated again, wondering what the heck I could say or do to get this student to focus. Jill was horsing around, not listening to anything I was saying. Her parents had paid a lot of money for me to be there for her birthday party, and I was afraid that I wouldn't be able to deliver value because she simply would not listen to my directions. In fact, Jill was not the first student to do this - it was a pattern that I'd noticed – only about one in every hundred children that I tried to teach would actually experience success. I attributed this success to their choosing to listen and follow my directions, and the failure of every other student to their refusal to do so.

Jill was having a great time, messing around and balancing the juggling balls on different parts of her body – head, neck, foot, back. Meanwhile, I was running out of time to get her juggling 3 balls. I was new at this business and I was trying to make a name for myself. The name I wanted to make wasn't "the guy who can't teach anyone to juggle". But I was so frustrated at the apparent lack of interest in almost **all** of my students to follow the technique. Didn't they realize that I was an expert? I'd travelled the world and performed for thousands, for heaven's sake!

The 3-ball cascade requires pretty strict adherence to technique, or it is impossible: time and accuracy are everything in technical juggling, and almost any sloppiness at all will make the whole pattern fall apart. Complex movements and near-perfect synchronization of visual and motor functions must happen several times every second without pause for even a 3-ball cascade to work.

As I was getting more and more worked up, Jill seemed not to notice or care – she was having a great time! Finally, as I was about to come down hard on her for not following my instructions, her mother came in, and was overjoyed to see her daughter having so much fun. I was puzzled – didn't she bring me here to get her daughter juggling? She turns to me and says:

"This is amazing! How did you get her to be so active? We struggle with this all the time, she just doesn't want to do anything physical. But look at this – she's getting so much exercise and we don't even have to pull her arm to get her to do it! What's your secret?"

In this moment, I had one of my most important discoveries about teaching. Until that point, I had been assuming that my own standards of success were the "correct" ones. That the 3-ball cascade was the only valid conclusion to reach in a juggling lesson. Taking a moment to watch Jill excitedly expressing herself in this new mode, and her overjoyed mother encouraging and celebrating her, I realized that I could not possibly call this lesson a failure.

After some more conversation with Jill's mother, I learned that Jill didn't generally like physical activity because she had a huge fear of being evaluated. Which is, unfortunately, exactly what children learn in school: Physical Education classes are
graded, and Jill never performed well. Jill hated phys. ed. classes because "all we do is play sports, and I'm not good at

sports". She had learned to hate physical activity because she was not successful at playing sports. Another huge definitions error with massive consequences for whole generations of students.

Defining physical activity only through the lens of competitive sports teaches millions of youth that physical activity is just not "for them". That's just as preposterous as assuming that you don't like music just because you wouldn't enjoy sitting through a 6-hour opera in a foreign language. But if that's your only access to music, how could you know any better?

From then on, I adjusted my goal: if I can encourage participation, self-expression, and empowering definitions of success, then I have done my job. More simply put, if they're taking part and having fun, then they're learning *something*. And really, who cares if that "something" is not the 3 ball cascade? What Jill needed was certainly not another judgemental and critical teacher with extremely narrow definitions of success. And there are **so many** Jills in the world who desperately need an alternative to being measured, evaluated, and pitted against their peers in competition. And if we don't give that to them, they'll live their whole lives with no compelling reason to engage in physical activity. The costs of this are monumental: emotionally, physically, financially (think healthcare costs) and fully avoidable if we can just change our definitions and our approach.

For students like Jill, a short juggling lesson with me may be the *only time* they get to experience success or the joy of being physical in a structured group activity. And for some, that's all it takes. In my case, one circus show inspired thousands of hours of learning, across more than a decade. I've seen students find a new way to define themselves, creating an identity that they're proud of, which they discovered and created through their pursuit of circus arts.

For the purposes of this book, I will define juggling as "Manipulating one or more objects in interesting ways." This does not necessitate throwing, catching, or for there to be a certain number of objects. It *does*, however, require that we depart from the normal ways that an object is used. If you use your spoon to eat, you are not juggling. But if you balance that spoon on your nose, I would consider that to be a kind of juggling. If you don't like my definition, no problem - get your own!

One last set of definitions to clarify before we jump in: Success, progress, and failure. I will define success as reaching an objective that we have set. It can change from person to person and from moment to moment. Progress involves actively taking steps toward anything (which can include "invisible" things like reading this book, pondering the subject, or talking about it), regardless of where those steps take us. Paths to success are so rarely straightforward, and it can be easy to get discouraged or give up when we perceive that we've "moved backwards". When building a sky-scraper, sometimes it takes months to build the foundation: if the structure's height is your only metric, you would be tempted to look at the hole in the ground and conclude that the builders are either incompetent or malicious. Don't get me wrong – metrics can sometimes be quite useful in assessing the effectiveness of our approach, but **not all progress is measurable, and not all measurements are useful**!

I'm going to spend a bit more time on failure because I believe that it's an important one to get clear. Failure, to me, is an attempt which does not achieve what you want to achieve. You have to try something, with a specific objective, and not achieve that objective. For example, if I wanted to build a shed, and what I built did not look or function like a shed, then I failed in that attempt. Even if my son decides it's a fun structure to play on and I decide to keep it, it would still be a failure to build a shed. Failure doesn't need to carry any implications at all with it (such as fault, shame, or blame)

Some say that the only true failure comes when you give up. I felt this way for a very long time. The only way that you can fail to juggle is to put the balls away and stop trying. But then I started a business as a new father, bit off more than I could chew, and giving up was one of the best decisions I've ever made. In fact, giving up can be a really important thing to do sometimes. Especially when the goal or the process no longer inspires you.

The hardest part of juggling is not teaching our hands the movements. That's actually fairly easy. The hard part is challenging our stories around it. We must learn to believe that it's possible, and that may require giving up a mindset that we've cultivated over years. We must also accept the certainty of making mistakes, which makes people uncomfortable. Making mistakes often carries with it criticism or the fear of criticism, which can be just as powerful an inhibitory force. When making mistakes or progressing at a slower pace than we'd hoped to, we need to keep a positive sense of self and separate our value as a person from our performance at the task.

I believe that juggling is a useful way to analyse how we relate to new tasks, drawing attention to the unseen processes that underly everything. When we do this, it allows us to notice and challenge our bad habits, to replace dysfunctional strategies with more effective ones, and to celebrate a return to childhood play. I encourage you to remember as you read this book: You are capable of so much more than you think!

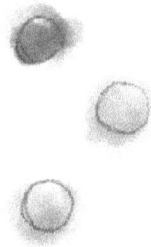

Part One:

Believe it's possible

Under Pressure

Years ago, I taught a juggling workshop at a local festival. There were a lot of families, and my juggling workshop station was one of the many activities that energetic kids could visit and hang out. We had a great time, playing and discovering the many joys of object manipulation. We had spinning plates, devilsticks, juggling balls, and a few other toys. At this point in my teaching career, I mostly taught by way of inviting and encouraging creative play, and then cheering on the results. You'd be amazed at how far students can come without actually having any technique-based teaching.

Our area was filled with laughter and joy, smiles, and cheers - we were immersed in the joy of play, discovery, and celebration. There wasn't a face in the room that wasn't sporting a huge smile. However, a new family joined us, looking rather somber. There was a boy around the age of 8, and a very stern-looking mother. I approached them and invited them to play with us - it looked like they needed it! When I run workshops at family events, it is typical for parents to leave their children with me and come back to collect them later - they rarely stay to participate.

After some prodding by the mother, the young boy very reluctantly stepped forward to collect the juggling balls I offered. I did my normal preamble, in which I explain the three rules of juggling using jokes and stories to lighten the mood and make participation seem a little less scary. As I talked, I noticed that the boy's anxiety was steadily mounting. He really didn't want to give it a try. When it came time to work on the first moves, the boy didn't begin. The mother, watching like a hawk, pounced on him and scolded him for his hesitation. She then proceeded to bully him quite forcefully to participate, when he clearly didn't want to.

The mood in the room changed tangibly. It was as if someone had cranked down an invisible energy dial for the activities. The kids who were happily playing began to notice the scolding mother and feel a little less free to express themselves. The boy looked quite upset, like he didn't want to be there at all. He kept asking to be done, but was forced to stay by his authoritarian mother. I was taken aback - this had never happened during one of my sessions. I wasn't sure what to do. I felt like asking this pushy mom to leave her kid alone and give him some space, but I didn't have enough confidence that I would know what to say or how to say it. So I did my best to counter her judgement and demands with celebration and encouragement.

It was clear though, that this was a terribly uncomfortable ordeal for the boy. I noticed that, on the rare occasions that he would try one of the moves I modelled, he only did so with the absolute bare minimum effort. He would then point out his failure and ask to be done: "Look, I can't do it! I can't! Can we leave now?"

Each time he "failed", his mother would become more stern and double down on her efforts to browbeat him into success. She got more and more flustered and frustrated and disappointed, until she reached her breaking point. She threw up her hands and said something pretty mean about her kid, and stormed away. He immediately relaxed, though he was obviously still feeling miserable about the exchange - he had just been scolded, bullied, and forced to embarrass himself in public, while being ridiculed for it by his mother. I did my best to try to re-frame the activity and help him experience a positive conclusion, but it was clear that he had had enough.

In that moment, I realized something pretty important - the boy had done this on purpose. He deliberately failed each try because that was the only strategy he had to get him out of the ordeal. He knew that if he frustrated his mother enough, she would finally get off his back and stop forcing him through this terrible trial. He probably was not consciously aware of what he was doing, but that's irrelevant - his actions were effective just the same. He did succeed in ending the trial, which was his primary goal - it was immensely distressing, and his actions were able to put a stop to it.

Whenever I approach any student, of any age, body type, of any ability or disability level, I always assume that they are capable of success. Almost every time, the students pick up on this assumption and act accordingly: "Oh, well, he probably wouldn't be asking me to do this if it was impossible. I'll trust that he is correct in his assessment of whether I can do this."

In this case, I saw that the mother did *not* have such a generous assumption - she assumed her boy would fail and that her responsibility was to hound him into success. In her paradigm, almost any amount of cajoling and cruelty would be justified, in order to achieve her goal of having a successful child (note that in her paradigm, *his* success belongs to *her* - she is *required to intervene constantly by pointing out mistakes and applying great psychological pressure*).

The problem is, the human brain doesn't work that way. Learning is considerably faster, more effective, and more enjoyable if we reinforce success rather than punish failure. When parents, educators, or peers treat us as if we will fail (unless they swoop in like heroes and rescue us with their grand wisdom and superiority), we learn to think of learning as a default-to-failure situation. That is, failure is the inevitable result, and only if we have access to just the right information or process or teacher, do we have any chance of succeeding. Not only does this type of parenting/teaching solidify the default-to-failure mindset in students, but it also makes students feel like garbage when they inevitably make mistakes.

When raised this way, children eventually internalize and carry with them this default-to-failure mindset, and it colours everything that they try (or don't try!). As a juggling instructor, it's clear as day to me - kids, in general, are happy to try new things like juggling. Adults, on the other hand, often make excuses and explicitly tell me that they are certain that they'll fail. In my opinion, this is because adults carry with them their own internal critic who watches closely and points out every failure and mistake.

This internal critic can be stupendously rude and judgemental, and poop on our parade so badly that it totally kills the mood. Not only does it kill the mood, but it fills us with anxiety, transforming what would otherwise be a joyous learning experience into a painful and dangerous trial by fire. And anyone with that internal critic (which is most people) knows that, once you've got it, it's nearly impossible to get rid of it. It's always there, watching and judging, with an endless supply of nasty things to say about us. It's no wonder that adults often hesitate to try new things! Especially things that can look silly when we mess up - like juggling!

Our anxiety around learning and making mistakes can make new endeavours feel too scary to try. Sometimes the anxiety grows so powerful that it even extends to things we can already do, and makes us feel like we can't or shouldn't do them. Things like grocery shopping, or talking to our neighbour. Sometimes it feels like it's so hard to face that it's easier to just avoid the anxiety altogether. If we could put a voice to the internal critic, it would tell us that our mistakes or our awkwardness are egregious and unforgivable. It would tell us that we can't do it, so we shouldn't even bother trying. Thus, we learn to shut down the possibility before we've even given it a fair chance. It is, after all, easier than having to face the anxiety of making mistakes and the almost-certain ridicule that we'll earn from our internal critic.

All this negative junk makes things feel so heavy that, like the boy in the story above, we can find ourselves deliberately failing in order to "prove" that we're not capable and so we shouldn't even be expected to try. I have found myself doing this on countless occasions - giving only a half-hearted try and then taking the expected failure as evidence that I should just quit. Perhaps you can think of times when you did the same thing. It's ok - we're all just human, and this is part of the package. We're just parroting the lessons that were given to us by well-meaning but misguided adults or peers. The good news is that we don't have to stay that way! Also part of being human is the ability to transcend our firmly held beliefs and change habits. Even if it's difficult.

Alright, let's get back on track here - we're talking about juggling, one of the most archetypally trivial and inconsequential activities that humans do. We're literally just picking up balls from the ground, doing a bunch of completely unnecessary things to them for our own amusement, and then putting them back where we got them. What does it even mean to "do it wrong"? It's not like someone is counting on the balls being in the air and will be let down if they're not. We're not transporting vital medical equipment to save lives. We're providing absolutely zero utility to the world. Functionally speaking, the stakes are as close to zero as it gets. In this context, it's almost comical how worked up we get about "doing it right", isn't it?

Juggling is perfect in that it provides us with a safe realm to investigate and tweak our assumptions about ourselves and how we relate to the tasks we perform.

When we remove the heaviness that we feel about learning, it becomes safe to try, and the process itself is incredibly rewarding. Feeling ourselves come alive is self-reinforcing. Once we feel it, we can never forget the experience.

We are so often worried that we are incapable that we render ourselves incapable. What we expect is what we get. But that unlimited potential stays in all of us, regardless of our ignoring or denying it. We have only to open up the possibility for it to exist, and it will. Greatness is built into us, as the potential to sprout is in every seed. There's just a whole lot that gets in our way and makes us forget.

I have found that it is pain and the fear of pain that keeps us from acknowledging our capabilities – like that time we tried and failed, and got cut down for trying. It's hard to believe that we do this to ourselves. In fact, we keep from ourselves even the awareness that we are doing it. Keeping ourselves protected, refusing to really *be* vulnerable and present and to learn. When asked, most of us wouldn't admit to doing it at all. We distract ourselves with all the pleasures, conveniences, and flashy things we can so that we don't have to face this internal rift. (when's the last time you made space to sit and think without a task at hand, for long enough to know what's really going on inside you?)

To be clear, I certainly don't mean to put myself in another category here – I'm just as guilty as the next person when it comes to protecting myself, refusing to try, and then blocking out all awareness that I am doing so. It has taken me almost 10 years to write this book *for that very reason!* I think that it's just as natural a part of us as is the ability to bloom and realize our potential. In fact, I try to think of our ability to deny our potential as proof of that very potential. Isn't it incredible how powerful our minds are? To think of how proficient we are at avoiding pain, blocking out the awareness that we are doing so (and keep up that façade 24/7) is incredible.

Another of the biggest barriers in acknowledging our capacities is the assumption that, **simply by admitting our capability to do something, we are also admitting our culpability in not doing that thing.** If we can achieve success, then *isn't it our fault for not doing so? What's wrong with us?* The consequent guilt and shame that comes up for us is often too painful to really look at, so we have to block our awareness of that question, pretend that we're not covering it up, and change the subject before it gets too uncomfortable. I want to be crystal clear here: By saying that you are capable of something, I am not meaning to say that you are responsible for doing that thing. It is your choice, and your choice alone whether you take advantage of your capabilities.

Actually, there are probably plenty of really good reasons for *not* learning, developing, and producing our best work. Apart from fear of failure, there may be people who count on you to maintain the status quo, who you feel you'd be abandoning if you really pursued something that's deeply meaningful to you. I know I find myself in that boat these days - between homeschooling my son and supporting my wife through full-time midwifery school, I definitely feel the weight of responsibility, and it's no joke!

I chose this life over one of potential personal fame and glory, because, to be frank, I find the standard definition of "success" to be self-centered and rather uncomfortable. In fact, it took quite a lot of work to create my own sense of what's meaningful that isn't just an echo of the very loudly proclaimed cultural goals of wealth, celebrity, and power. After a great deal of work, I am now able to simultaneously acknowledge my capacity to become a highly successful juggler, businessperson, or fill-in-the-blank, and decide that I don't want to. I have chosen to explore instead whether the two sets of priorities can coexist, while trying to confront all of the deep (and often invisible) roadblocks that get in the way.

I say all of this to convey that *I have struggled for years with the guilt of "I can, therefore I should".* It takes deep knowledge of self and profound clarity of purpose and priority to be able to admit that we are capable without also feeling the compulsion to exercise those capabilities. Much easier to just bury the whole package and forget about it.

Alright, enough philosophizing - time for an activity! You can do this for real or just as a hypothetical - whatever you've got the courage for!

Cold Showers (AKA - "Dear God, No!")

What if I told you that taking cold showers drastically improves your health? What if you could kick that nasty cold weeks earlier? Or, even better, not get it in the first place? Cold showers are great for fat loss, improving immune function, and even make your hair look nicer. No, I'm not making this up – there's actually evidence for each of these points. But here's the kicker – you have to actually **do it.** *You have to turn the dial all the way to cold, interrupt your nice, soothing, warm shower to sputter and gasp at the shock of the cold, and do the cold dance while trying not to slip and break your neck. Yes, even in the* *middle of winter.*

Doesn't sound very pleasant, does it? Well, do you think you can do it? I'll bet your answer is a resounding "no way!" Most people HATE the cold. In fact, even people who struggle with continuous illness (I'm talking about coughs, colds, and flus, not cancer), who swear up and down that they'll try anything, still stop short of cold showers. "Uh-uh, no WAY Andrew, I can't do that! Not in a million years!"

So what's the holdup, exactly? It's obviously not going to kill you. It will be unpleasant (sometimes profoundly so) for about 30 seconds, and afterward it tends to feel pretty exhilarating. You know, endorphins and all that good stuff. So what gets in the way? Perhaps there's not sufficient motivation? Sure, it takes a whole lot of willpower to turn that dial, I won't deny that. But there's a whole world of difference between "can't" and "don't want to".

What about places in the world where they don't HAVE the luxury of hot water? Showers are cold by default. Would you never clean yourself? I'll bet that if you were covered in some caustic liquid that was about to dissolve your flesh, that cold shower would feel pretty appealing, wouldn't it?

I bring up cold showers as an easy example that most people can identify with, but it may or may not resonate with you. I'm almost certain that there are lots of examples of things that you do this with, for one reason or another. Perhaps you feel that something is too risky to consider. Rock climbing or other "dangerous" activities (side note: rock climbing is actually statistically quite safe. You are far more likely to get injured playing badminton.) often don't show up on our list of fun things to do because we believe we can't.

Maybe for you it's a career aspiration (I always wanted to try music/drawing/fill-in-the-blank…). Perhaps it's about vulnerability in the context of a relationship ("I could never be myself here, he/she would be horrified to know who I am on the inside!"). Or maybe it's something that you have no awareness at all that you're even doing ("I'd love to meet this famous person, but they'd never want to talk to me…"). I have found that we are willing to stamp a big, indelible "I CAN'T" onto many things that we've never tried before, and it can be shocking when we really come to see how many opportunities we deny ourselves by doing this.

So, Andrew, is all of this just to make me change my words from "I can't" to "I don't want to"?!

Well, yes! With the utmost respect, I don't really care whether you want to, or choose to, do something challenging such as juggling. What I *do* care about is when you tell yourself that you can't. Why do I care? Well, 'cause it's downright disrespectful! I would feel insulted if you told *me* that I couldn't learn to do something. I would also feel insulted if you said that about a friend or family member, just as I feel insulted when you say it about yourself.

Believing that you are capable of whatever it is that's in front of you is a foundation of respect that we all deserve from ourselves. Without that foundation, any learning can become too risky, and we come to live in cages that we've built for ourselves, simply because it's too scary to venture outside. Like renouncing the use of your legs just because you might fall sometime. If you think I'm being dramatic, bear with me.

You'll never know the extent of the cost you pay by denying your capabilities. First, because you're usually unaware that you're doing it, and second, because you can't know what benefits come from things if you don't learn them. Refusing to even look at a map of a place you've never been means that you'll never learn what richness exists there. Not to mention that you signal to others around you that it's ok to sell yourself short. Who's watching you when you do this? Your kids? Maybe your students? Co-workers? Partners? This kind of stuff spreads, you know! On the plus side, so does courage, and telling the truth (For example: "Actually, I could quite easily turn the dial to cold on my shower, I just don't want to!")

In the end, whether you're willing to take on this model is up to you. If you experience hesitation or resistance to accepting my words, then I would challenge you to ask yourself: why? What's the harm in believing the best of yourself? You probably can't put your finger on it, maybe you just feel a sense of unease. If so, great! That's completely normal. When we push the boundaries of our models, a sense of unease or discomfort is our natural response. But guess what? You're capable of weathering that storm too! How do I know? Because I've walked so many people through this process before. Not to mention that I've gone through the process personally more times than I can count.

If it's too much and you really can't bring yourself to believe something is possible, at the very least, **suspend your disbelief.** Push pause on that narrative in your head that's trying to tell you that you can't do something. Devote a small chunk of time to simply exploring whether something *could be possible.* Do some research before making a conclusion! Science!

> *In fact, let's try it right now. It's Juggling Time! Flip to the end of the book and follow exercise one for just five minutes, and come on back.*

Well, can you juggle now?

Even if the answer is "no, I still can't juggle", at least then you'll actually know. Actually, that's incorrect. A more accurate statement would be "I can't juggle *yet.*" Or, "I can't juggle after 30 seconds of distracted and unmotivated attempts".

Oh come on, let's be honest. *If* you actually put the book down and tried it (Yeah, I was watching, I saw you totally not do it), it wasn't really your best effort, was it? If you didn't do it already, go ahead. I'll wait right here.

Did you do it this time? If you did and it worked, great! You just proved that you are capable achieving something new! If it *still* didn't work, I'll ask you this: What if I told you that we've run out of oxygen and oxygen is only being given out to people who can juggle? I'll bet you'd learn real quick then, wouldn't you! An absurd example, of course, but if you still have trouble believing, ask yourself this: If I had enough motivation, do I truly doubt that I would be able to learn how to juggle? If my life depended on it?

YOU are capable of _____

For most people, believing this is the hardest point to achieve. For some, telling them that they're capable of juggling is like telling them they're capable of human flight. It seems so absurd and farfetched that they don't even know how to object. Though, of course, that doesn't stop them (from objecting, I mean). I've done this long enough that I've heard every excuse in the book. Things like "I can't – I'm too clumsy." "I drop things all the time." Someone even said to me once: "I can't even tie my own shoelaces!" What? This was from a teenager, by the way, who was in fact, fully capable of tying her own shoes.

The power of not making excuses

I'd like to share with you the story that I begin each juggling workshop with. Years ago, I taught a boy named Anthony. Anthony was a remarkable kid, for several reasons. One was that he was born missing half of his left arm. The bottom half, in case you're wondering. On his right hand, he was missing his thumb, index finger, and half of his middle finger. That left him with the weak half of only one hand. I knew that this was something I needed to play carefully – I had no way of knowing how he related to his body until we started the workshop. As per my default, I decided to approach Anthony with the assumption that he would be able to juggle if he chose to, just like everyone else in the room.

And sure enough, Anthony blew me away with his spirit. He didn't breathe a word of complaint about the difficulty of juggling without the tools that most of us take for granted.

Instead, he spent the time exploring the things that he was able to do. By the end of the workshop, he was able to juggle two balls in his one hand, with minor support in catching and stabilising from his other arm. He was a star, and the rest of the kids at the workshop went ballistic when they saw what Anthony was able to achieve.

Anthony may not have known it at the time, but I believe that what he was performing was, in fact, magic. I define magic as anything that contradicts our sense of what's possible. Magic forces us to suspend our disbelief and expand our idea of what's possible. His audience watched with jaws dropped, their assumptions of Anthony (and themselves) shattered.

I have worked with all manner of people before, including those with physical, intellectual, and social disabilities, and what I've learned is that if there's a will, there's a way. When a person spends their time testing what IS possible, there's no time for what's not possible. And the act of exploring those limits is empowering – the more vigorously we challenge our assumed limitations, the more pliable they become.

What it looks like

So what does this rule look like in practice? I can explain it all I want, but I believe that an experience will be much more valuable for you. In my current life as a workshop facilitator, I use a game to bring awareness to our self-talk around possibility/impossibility. If you'd like to try it, be my guest!

The paper game

Here's a fun game you can play that probably won't take much time. I'd recommend that you actually try it, even if you only spend a minute or two on it. It provides you with a valuable perspective that is difficult to imagine without going through the motions.

Materials:
- **Paper (any size).** *What's that? You don't have any paper? I don't believe you – you're holding a great big bunch of paper in your hands this very moment! Don't worry, I won't be offended if you rip the book. Flip to the appendix for a couple of sample pages.*
- **Scissors (optional).** *They will make the game easier, but if you can rip carefully, you can play with just your hands.*

Goal: *to cut/tear a hole in the piece of paper that you can pass your entire body through. And before you go off on some clever solution (don't get me wrong – I love creative solutions!), I'll clarify: the object is quite literal. It's not a play on words: you must actually pass your entire physical body through the hole! The hole must be contained within a continuous border -*

No tape or joining of ends!

Side note - when my wife first presented me with this game, I cut a chunk out of the paper, wrote the words "my entire body" on it, and passed it through the hole. She informed me that I was smartass, and needed to find the actual solution. I won't call you a smartass, but you get the point.

Ready.... Go!

Debrief:
When you've given it a good try, and feel like you're finished, let's discuss how it went. Some of the questions I like to ask participants of this game are:

- *How did it go?*
- *Did you succeed in making a hole big enough for your body to pass through?*
- *What were your thoughts or feelings as you played the game?*
- *Did you find yourself saying "This is impossible"? If so, how did your assessment affect your actions?*

For the record, I don't think that it matters much whether you succeeded in this game or not. The reason I presented the challenge is so that you can get a snapshot of how you react to seemingly-impossible challenges. I believe that the way you reacted to this game is probably the same as how you react to a lot of things in your life.

The vast majority of participants react to this game by loudly declaring that it's impossible, folding their arms across their chests, and refusing to take any action at all. Without venturing into the unknown, they sit back and look around the room at other people's efforts, sometimes criticising, sometimes silent, but almost always without challenging their initial narrative.

After all, once people have heard you say that it's impossible, how can you justify making any effort at all?

By the way, please note that I bring no judgement with that question. I can't possibly tell you that if you gave up and stopped trying, it's a bad thing. I can only decide what's good for me. It's up to you to decide your values. I only gave you that exercise to allow you to observe yourself. Whether you're happy with your approach or not is up to you!

One final point before we move on: this game is admittedly pretty trivial in that it doesn't matter if you gave up or not. But can you say the same about every other situation you bring your assessments and choices into?

(In case you're curious, it IS, in fact, possible. And no, I'm not telling you how.)

...Ok, fine, here's a hint: there's two ways, and both of them involve making the paper into a big, long, coiled strip.

Good luck!

So how do we practice this principle?

I believe that it begins with creating space in between a possibility and our judgment of that possibility. When a random stranger shows up with a unicycle and suggests that you can learn how to ride it, it means *not* responding with an immediate "I can't". It is the shifting of our perspective from teacher to student. Rather than "knowing" and having to convince everyone that you "can't" do something, be an inquisitive student of your abilities.

Ask questions rather than making statements. Ask yourself "Can I?" "IS this possible for me?" "Do I *want to* do this? And if not, why not? How can I be certain that this is 'too risky'?" "What do I actually **know** (as opposed to feel) about this?"

In practice, setting your self-belief meter's default to "I can" rather than "I can't" is not about arrogance. It's about allowing for possibilities, not proclaiming superiority. It's about allowing "I can" to be possible by not shutting it out. Again, it's about studying and exploring rather than proclaiming.

To use a gardening analogy, become a great gardener! Plant the seeds of possibility and then care for and protect them. Things will only grow and bloom if you plant them. That means doing things that matter to you. If you value your health, *try* a cold shower! (note that this is not medical advice, and don't sue me…) If you value singing, take a class in it! If you have a wacky and wild business idea, draft a simple plan! Plant the seeds and see what grows. Some will and some won't, but you'll never know if you don't believe it's possible and try.

Another helpful tip: *believe in others!* When we hold generous assumptions of others' capabilities, they will often rise to them. Sometimes they'll grumble about it, but they'll often take advantage of the support. To give a great example of this, my 6-year-old son Lewis cooks dinner for the family once a week. Most people can't believe this, but it's true. In fact, I believe that we started him on it when he was 3 years old. The meals may not be very sophisticated (it's pretty much always pasta with pesto and chopped veggies), but that's not important. What's important is that he has risen to the challenge so many times that this is now a deeply-ingrained part of his worldview.

You'll find that generous assumptions can be the lead domino that creates a whole cascade of changes down the line. How will Lewis's life be different over the coming decades when he brings with him the knowledge that he can cook? (I can't help but compare this with my adult friends who still don't have confidence that they can cook). How about the knowledge that he can solve problems and figure things out? That he can take risks and learn new things? How does *your* life look when you hold these beliefs? What cascade of possibilities would *you* explore if you knew deep down that you were capable?

When it goes wrong

So what causes us to make unfavourable conclusions about ourselves and the world? Why do we end up with the idea that we *can't* do something? I believe that there are a few reasons:

• **When we genuinely try something a whole bunch and it doesn't work out**

As children, we are avid experimenters. We're constantly testing things to learn more about how the world works and how it doesn't work. Watch a small child sometime, and notice how many times they try things. Everyone has their own degree of persistence, but you'll notice that once a child tries the same thing several times and it doesn't work out, they move on to the next thing. Of course they do – that's what learning is, isn't it? If we didn't learn this, we'd still be trying to balance a round ball on top of another round ball, only to have it continue to fall off.

So what do we do? We draw the conclusion that this is impossible, and we move on. This is a really important stage in learning – making conclusions and altering our future actions in accordance with our new rule. The problem? Despite our best efforts, we're not always correct when we write the rules in our mental rulebook, and we generally don't like to revisit them. It feels challenging to our ego to confront the possibility that our carefully curated rulebook has errors. As it turns out, there are a few ways to balance a round ball on top of another round ball – changing the shape of the balls, glueing them together, or (my favourite), spinning the balls around their central axis.

• **When we set our definitions such that success is impossible**

When we set the bar so high that it looks impossible, we can't help but quit before we've begun. Seeking to achieve tasks that we believe deep down to be impossible is a fool's errand, and we simply won't try. This can also be a wise thing to do: in a world of limited resources, why would we waste them on things that are (in our minds) unachievable? If you ask me to jump off a cliff and fly away, I would correctly state that this is impossible and decline to participate in the challenge. Again, why would I waste my limited resources (in this case, my life) on something that I believe to be impossible?

Using an absurd example like jumping off a cliff makes it obvious, but it's rarely so in real life. Our culture is terrible for its propagation of unachievable standards. There's a frantic drive to have it all and do it all – not only do we feel immense pressure to be employed and make ever more money, but it has to be something deeply meaningful that will change the world. Not only do we need to have a romantic partner, but we need to be fully compatible with them in every way, they need to be an exemplary human being and also beautiful and similarly employed. We need to have a house, but not just any house – it needs to be nice and in a good location, recently renovated, etc. I could go on and on, but I think you get the point.

If you set out to do something new, don't set your bar for success so high! That's like imagining that the first step of a marathon should be across the finish line. There's a whole lot that has to come in between! Actually, that's where the richness comes in. Can you imagine if achieving the superlative level of success in any domain happened instantly upon your first try? How boring and meaningless would *everything* become if that were the case?

Here's a story from my time in the circus about how much we're truly capable of, and how suspending the expectations of our performance can sometimes allow us to exceed ourselves in unexpected ways.

Worst Circumstances = Best Work?

"I need all hands on the tent RIGHT NOW!!!"

Poles crashed to the ground, walls buckled and fell. We've been working over 24 hours now with no sleep. In that moment, any lack of sharpness or misstep could have meant death. That was about the time when the jet planes started taking off about 40 feet from our circus tent...

Let me back up and give a little context to this story. It's the summer of 2008, somewhere around July 3rd. I'm touring England in the Festival Circus, working as a juggler, acrobat, and unicyclist. It was one of the more unique experiences I've had: I was simultaneously a student of the Academy of Circus Arts and a performer in the Festival Circus, which were one and the same. I like to think of that troupe as some kind of superhero – to the public, we were The Festival Circus, but our secret identity was that we were a bunch of students at the Academy of Circus Arts. I kept a journal in the small scraps of time I had available, so as not to lose the great stories to the mists of time, or to my leaky memory.

That summer was many things, one of which I'm sure now was a scam: we paid many thousands of dollars for the privilege of doing some of the hardest work on the planet without pay for months on end, performing to make the owner money. I say this in jest – I don't think the owner made any money at all. Also, it was certainly the most profound and valuable formative experience of my life. In just 6 months, we performed 135 shows in 25 locations across the UK. This was probably the hardest time of my life, and also the time where I grew most and did some of my best work. I'm sharing this story to illustrate the point of how we can often do our best work in the worst circumstances. Now, back to the story:

The previous day, we rose at 6:00 AM in Whitehaven, toward the North end of England. We had to pack up the tent (which seats approx. 700 people) and drive across the country to our next location at a private airport in London for Employee Day. Packing up the tent on a good day, with a crew of 18 hard workers working at a full sprint without breaks, takes 3-4 hours plus 30-60 minutes for the bleachers. We were short-handed and had just finished a long string of shows, so we were pretty tired for the wake-up call at 6:00 AM. We managed to finish by noon, and head out for London. It was a beautiful drive on a beautiful summer day, through a gorgeous countryside. It felt like nothing could go wrong. We were supposed to arrive at 8:00 PM, but as things typically go in the circus, we ran into many problems and didn't arrive until about 10:00 PM.

Now, we were told that this would be a really difficult gig, as we had to build up the tent overnight, only sleep a couple of hours, and then do 7 full shows back-to-back with no real breaks. We were also told that the airport security would be prepared for our arrival and able to assist us in our setup by providing water, food and coffee, bathroom access, etc. This was false.

The reception we got from security was anything but warm or helpful. In fact, they seemed to be operating under the instructions to harass, interfere, delay, and irritate us. It started with their refusing to let us onto the runway, where we were supposed to build the tent. They told us that this would be impossible, and it was only after about 3 hours of reviewing our contract and the explicit communications with the organizers that they reluctantly let us into the compound (with aggressive pat-downs of everyone in our troupe, of course).

Now it's after midnight, and we have less than 9 hours to set up our tent on an airport runway without driving a single stake into the ground. Normally setting up a tent this size requires driving in over 100 solid iron stakes, weighing in at 35 pounds each, to a depth of about 4 feet. To make matters worse, we're also at about half our normal crew size – some vehicles broke down along the way, as was common (circuses are often quite poor and can't afford good vehicles), and 3 of the students were severely injured. One threw out her back that morning, another, our contortionist, injured one of her major nerves from overstretching, and was hospitalized. The third had the tightwire frame collapse on and break her foot, and the icing on the cake came when we found out that she was *allergic to the painkillers and was not only in agonizing pain, but also vomiting all over the site. Security, needless to say, was not amused... By 3:30 AM, we had to call an ambulance, and buildup had only just begun.*

One of the vehicles that hadn't arrived yet was my bunkwagon, so I didn't have any of my work clothes or anything. So there I was, standing on this windy airport runway in the middle of the night, freezing cold in shorts, undershirt and sandals, being harassed by obnoxious security guards, while trying to do the work of two to three people in half the time, knowing that I've got a full day of shows ahead.

By 4:30 AM, the sandbags (which we used to anchor the tent) were finally set, and we could start actually building the tent. I don't think that I've ever worked faster or harder in my life. The 8 or so of us that made up the crew that night were labouring like maniacs under the desperate hope that, if we got the tent built in time, we might have an hour to lay down before our shows start. 5:00 arrives and we pause for ten seconds to admire the beautiful pink sunrise before returning to work. By 6:30, my bunkwagon finally arrives along with 2 more workers. I haven't eaten anything now since noon the previous day. Our crew stops for 5 minutes to scarf down as much food as we possibly can and get right back to work.

It's now 7:00 AM, the tent is built, and we need to do 3 hours more work setting the seating, lights, sound, curtain, props, and ring, before our shows start at 9:00. We're panicking. We all jump out to the seating trailer and start to unload the bleachers. The sight we saw at that moment still haunts me. A jet plane rounds the corner and is about to take off. On the runway. Directly beside our tent.

Now, if you've ever set up a circus tent in high winds, you know that it's essentially just a GIANT oversized kite that would happily fly away if given the chance. The bleacher frames clatter soundlessly to the ground amid the roar of the engines as we stand in shock while the plane picks up speed toward the tent. Time is moving in slow motion. The plane is not. Surely, they knew that we were going to have a tent here, right? They booked us months in advance. No one is so incompetent that they didn't make this connection, right? ...Right?!

None of that matters in the moment. We stand frozen as the plane flies by at takeoff speed and the tent objects in the strongest possible terms. Our work is being undone before our eyes as the poles fall and the walls and ceiling start to crumple inward.

"I need all hands on the tent RIGHT NOW!!!" Our director and legendary circus instructor Ann Dorwin shouts at us. We're snapped out of our paralysis and rush into the tent as it is collapsing, picking up poles and striving inhumanly to restore the structure before the whole thing falls in and crushes us. It was one of the scariest moments of my life – people have died in tent collapses in circus history. The danger wasn't abstract, it was real, and our ability to make good decisions was held up only by our adrenaline after over 24 hours of work.

That was the first of the 4 planes that took off that morning, and each time we had to drop everything and attend to the tent. Luckily, no one died, though it wasn't for lack of trying on the part of this cursed airport. As you may have guessed, we had less than zero time for sleep or rest before our first show.

I had run out of water halfway through the trip the previous day and was looking pretty shabby from all the work. I had to shave, but the airport security absolutely would not let us into the building. So I had to shave with a bowl of orange juice. Yes, I actually did that. Razorburn, anyone? I then had to put makeup on my sticky face, and perform 7 back-to-back shows of 75 minutes, with zero breaks in between (all gaps were filled with the work we hadn't been able to do before we started our shows). At precisely 8:00 PM when our last show was finished, security wasted no time at all in reminding us that we were not welcome and were to pack up and leave. Immediately. And no, they weren't going to help.

We finished at 2:00 AM, and managed to pull all of our vehicles out of the airport and across the street to an empty parking lot. We weren't able to rest or sleep until the last vehicle arrived at 3:00AM (they had been stranded, broken down on the side of the road halfway across the country this whole time). We had just finished a marathon of 45 hours of the most intense work without sleep. The punchline – half of our troupe was homeless this entire time because the last vehicle to join us was one of the bunkwagons. That meant that they had no access to any of their clothing, personal items, or even toilets – we had to share ours.

You might have thought that the shows we put on would be terrible. I would have thought that too. But I would have been wrong. In fact, they were the best shows that I had done to date. Why? At the time, I thought that it was because I didn't care if the audience liked it or not. My anxiety level around doing a good show was as close to zero as you can get. The result was that I wasn't worried about dropping while I juggled, and so I didn't. I had no expectations that things would go well, so I didn't have to keep comparing reality to my story. I didn't have the time or the energy to self-evaluate. I was simply there with the audience, in that moment, with no expectations or story to come between us. In short, I was fully present. And the audience recognized that. They would never have guessed what we'd been through.

The audience never knew our story. Even if they had, I don't think they would have cared. They came to see a show and all that we had been through was irrelevant to them. All of the stuff that makes our work difficult doesn't matter to the audience – and it's never an excuse to give any less than our best. I learned that all these stories we keep in our heads just come between us and our audience. As we were told by Ann, "the show must go on", and as long as we're still standing, we have a duty to deliver.

The most inspiring teachers, leaders, and performers I've ever known let their struggles energize rather than drain them. In fact, in my life as an entrepreneur, a business mentor once gave me an incredibly valuable piece of advice when he said "you'll never have a life without struggle. You just have to choose the struggles that make you grow and feel invincible." Whenever I start to consistently resent my struggles, I take it as a sign that I'm in the wrong line of work.

I think that sometimes our problems can become blessings if we let them. Minor setbacks can often stress us out because we're still trying to keep our work on track. But when things reach a critical level of messed up, and our plans get mangled *beyond repair, we can no longer kid ourselves about it. We then have to step out of our stories and deal with reality – we have to be present with what is, rather than what we planned or wished. Our plan to set up in time to be able to sleep was smashed to bits. We encountered a dozen problems we never thought we'd have to deal with – like the razorburn that comes from shaving with orange juice. And in the end we had to laugh as we threw our plans in the garbage and did our exhausted best to give the audience a good time.*

Luckily, we had the best director on the planet, a great troupe of hard workers, and a great team dynamic. The result was that we laughed a lot. And I mean a LOT. Problems stacked up so high that we couldn't even count them anymore. There are at least a dozen incidents that didn't even make it into this story, for brevity's sake. That summer, I learned that we are capable of so much more than we think, and our expectations only get in the way. As any parent knows, you stretch to meet the demands of a new human life, no matter the cost. Sometimes it takes a tragedy, an accident, or just a totally sideways and unexpected event to take us out of our heads and to let us learn what we're truly capable of.

Remember, when you think you're at your end, you may only just be beginning...

As a final note, when the organizers learned of our struggles and saw how honestly we gave ourselves in the ring, they invited us back next year for double the pay and the promise of a better plan for security. We gained a reputation as a one-in-a-million troupe who would give everything in service of our clients.

Sometimes we wait until the circumstances are right before acting, but my experience is that we are woefully ignorant of what circumstances we actually need to do our best work. The story you just read is a great example of the supreme importance of our inner circumstances over our outer circumstances. If you can get into the right frame of mind (which includes mindful and realistic goal-setting), you'll find that you can surprise yourself with what you're capable of.

Maybe that's the key – to have your excellent performance come as a surprise to you by not expecting it as the default. And you don't have to believe you'll experience a bad outcome to make this possible – you simply drop your stories of how it's going to turn out.

And lastly,

- **When we get constant messages from others that we're not capable**

I think that this is frighteningly common, and very unfortunate. In fact, I would argue that it's a favourite cultural pastime these days. Think of how immensely successful our current talent competitions are: American Idol, So You Think You Can Dance, America's Got Talent. The entire premise of these shows is to judge and reject people until there's no one left to judge and reject, with the last person standing being revered as some kind of god. Judges are not always very kind in their feedback – as with any mass media, these shows thrive on emotional engagement, and it's so damn easy to manipulate audiences. For whatever reason, people think it's fun to collectively mock those who aren't good at singing, dancing, or whatever they've come to do. As viewers, what's the lesson we walk away with? "Wow, I sure am glad I'm not *that guy!* At least I **know** that I can't sing!"

We eventually internalize the message that mistakes are to be mocked, until we stop trying.

And if we haven't gotten the message yet, our friends, parents, educators try to "help" us by making sure that we remember. We're constantly being given messages of prudence, risk aversion, and "playing it safe". This was the very thought my parents had when they suggested in no uncertain terms that I **not** pursue a career in circus arts. They had nothing but love and concern in their hearts, for which I can't fault them. But the resulting message was far less than helpful. In fact, I feel like I owe all of the richness that's in my life right now to the risks that I took. And if I had listened to the messages of concerned onlookers, I would never have taken those crucial first steps.

When we spend our time remarking on the mistakes or limitations of others, we are secretly doing the same thing to ourselves. Eventually, no one even needs to criticize us because we learn to do it to ourselves.

When you say "I can't", it may have a lot of baggage and past experience attached to it. I understand - being chastised for mistakes hurts, and that memory gets burned into our brains so that we don't forget. Acknowledging our capabilities means confronting those past experiences and letting go of them.

To use a metaphor, if your hands are full of memories, there's no room to put the juggling balls! In short, the same working space we use for innovation and risk-taking can get filled up with painful emotional baggage. Coming to terms with the possibility of making mistakes is ultimately important in taking the risk of believing in what's possible. We'll talk more in the next chapter about how to do this.

Coming back

It's ok to drop the ball on this one. As we saw, there are many reasons why we forget this lesson, and none of them are our "fault". I'd like to talk about a few ways that we can come back to practicing this rule.

First, I'd like to explore the importance of our choice of language. When we say that we can't do something, it sounds pretty final, doesn't it? Just listen: "I can't". There's nowhere to go from there, is there? It's a dead-end sentence that creates a dead-end for our learning. What we're essentially saying with this choice of words is:
- I cannot do _____ at this moment
- Therefore, I shouldn't even bother trying: I'll **never** be able to do _____

When I hear my students say this, I invite them to tack on a more promising ending: "I can't juggle… yet!" This revised statement is an invitation to realize our potential rather than a closed door that allows no other possibility. Even if we never learn to juggle, the statement remains true. When we change our language, it can have a profound impact on our thoughts.

To give an example of this in action, I'll tell a story.

Piece of Cake!

During my initial inspiration of learning to juggle, I would find myself attempting very difficult skills such as a 5-ball 5-up pirouette. In plain English, that means juggling 5 balls, throwing all 5 of them up very high, spinning your body in a full circle, and then catching the balls as they come down and continuing the juggling pattern.

With all of the failure I was experiencing, I found myself saying in my head "Ah, jeez! This is so hard!", which became "I'll never be able to get this!" and then "this trick is impossible!". That's right, I'm not immune to this human habit!

In fact, it felt like these statements were just summing up reality. I had tried it a hundred times in a row and I still didn't feel any closer, so that meant this trick was hard or even impossible. If it were a scientific experiment, I was drawing conclusions based on the evidence I was gathering. Look: it's obviously impossible because, even though I'm a good juggler, I can't do this even after weeks of practice. I'm not selling myself short, my beliefs are grounded in evidence!

What I eventually noticed was how frustrating this whole experience was. I had been a learning machine up to that point! I learned so much, why was it stopping now? Had I finally reached my limit? Why can I do almost the same thing (a 5-ball 3-up pirouette: throwing three and holding two during the spin) but not this one? Is it a hard stop at a 3-up? That seemed ridiculous, but it also seemed true – no matter how many times I tried, I just couldn't get it!

*In the spirit of play, I decided to try things a little bit differently. Rather than letting the stories I was telling (such as "this is hard" or "I can't do this") go unchecked in my head, I decided to challenge them. Even though it **felt** like those were factual statements, I decided to defy them just to see what would happen.*

In my next practice session, I started smiling every time I tried the trick and saying in my head "this trick is a piece of cake". I'll be honest – I felt like a real idiot. I even started forcing myself to say it out loud: "Ah, piece o' cake!" I did this over and over again, no matter how spectacularly I failed.

I knew it was absurd, but I stuck with it. And you probably already know what happened next. I started to make some progress. Very slowly, I started catching more of the balls. One day, I actually got the trick, and I was over the moon with excitement.

After that, the habit stuck. Whatever new skill I was trying to get, I would repeat my mantra: "piece of cake... piece of cake...". People would sometimes give me weird looks, but I didn't let that stop me. I just had the confidence that I would eventually prove that I could do it. And even if I couldn't, I would be confident that I had given it my actual best.

There's a saying that I once heard, and it seems to sum this up perfectly:

"Whether you believe you can, or whether you believe you can't: you're right."

The power of the mind is absolutely incredible. We are capable of so much that I believe that most of us will never discover the vast majority of what we're capable of within our lifetimes. We make assessments about what's possible that *seem* factual, but sometimes those definitions are more permeable than we think.

The Power of Stories

Here's a little micro-experiment for you to try. You can do it next time you really have to pee but you're not near a toilet. Or in that final, Olympic-speed run for the toilet/urinal/ nearest tree, I want you to try something. Tell yourself "I don't have to pee. Nah, it's fine, I could wait. No big deal." You have to actually mean it though. **Act as if** *that's true. Walk slowly. Let someone ahead of you.*

In my experience, it seems like a switch flips, and even though I still have the feeling, it loses all of its urgency. I suspect that it is the contrast between our first story (Oooh! Havetopeehavetopeehavetopeerealbad!) and our second story (I'm totally fine waiting to pee) that constructs our experience and the consequent sense of, or lack of, urgency.

One last factoid that I'd like to share: Did you know that everybody in Japan learns to ride a unicycle? It's true! In grades 3 and 4, students are taught to ride unicycles in their physical education classes: it's part of school curriculum. When I tell people this, it's often met with disbelief. It's hard for this fact to coexist with the assumption that riding a unicycle is "impossible", or that it requires some particular talent that few people are blessed with. I think that these assumptions are born from the scarcity of unicyclists in North America. You can see how easy it is to assume that, if you only see one person ride a unicycle out of the millions of people you've ever seen, you could conclude that only one in a million people *can* ride a unicycle. And if only one in a million can ride one, it must be exceptionally difficult!

I believe that we all make our assessments of what's possible and what's impossible based on what we're exposed to. Of course we do! That's what learning is: we observe the world around us, and then we make rules to explain why things are the way that they are, and apply those rules to predict how they'll be in the future. We base all of our decisions and beliefs on these rules that we've internalized. This is a very powerful mechanism that allows us to adapt to and make good functional decisions about how to act. There is nothing wrong with this process – we're actually very good at it.

However, things become problematic when we don't get exposed to things that expand our worldview. And when we eventually *do* encounter those things that defy our previous understanding of the world, we can be pretty reluctant to revise our model to incorporate this new information. It's much easier to just sweep it under the rug and pretend it doesn't exist, or to justify or explain it in some way.

It can be quite difficult to adjust the models by which we understand the world because, in some sense, it makes us wrong. In order to incorporate new information, we have to be willing to confront the fact that we've made an error (or even that our model was incomplete), and that can sometimes feel like it's too much.

Coming to terms with our mistakes can be an incredibly difficult undertaking, especially for those of us who were raised with shame. That is, the idea that **we ought to be embarrassed about our mistakes** – that mistakes are proof of some fundamental flaw in who we are. We are such good learners that, when we are shamed for our mistakes, we learn to shame ourselves. Shame transforms mistakes into harbingers of doom, which we must fear and avoid at all costs. We learn that mistakes call into question our value as human beings, and the fear of making mistakes grows into an existential terror. We learn to live our lives confined to the things that we can already do well and avoid areas of growth, as we know that they will cause us to make mistakes and experience deep pain.

The trouble is that we lose out on so much when we live this way - our mistakes are not only incredible teachers, but also the source of some of our richest experiences. In fact, I don't believe that learning itself is possible without mistakes. Mistakes are so important that the next chapter is dedicated to them.

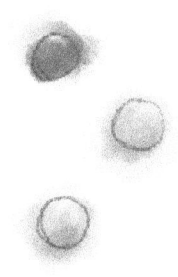

Part Two:

Drop the ball

BZZZZT! WRONG!

Have you ever played Operation? You know, the game where you have to wield tweezers with extreme precision in order to remove things like a Charlie Horse or Funny Bone from a dopey-looking goof with a big red nose that lights up when you make a mistake? Well, I have. I have a very strong memory of the game. In fact, it's one of the few things I remember well from my childhood.

Now, you might think that, as a professional juggler who has set world records for dexterity and coordination, I'd have been good at this game. However, this was not the case. In fact, when I was introduced to the game, I think I was too young to have either the dexterity or the emotional maturity to play. Sounds funny, but I think that Operation exposes an important feature of our psyche - how we relate to mistakes.

In case you've never played the game, let me explain: You have to use a tiny set of tweezers to remove strangely shaped objects out of corresponding strangely shaped holes in the patient (who is a 2-d character reclined on an operating table). There is very little clearance between the objects and the very small holes from which they are to be removed, and if your tweezers touch the edge even for a split second, the game board lights up and a very loud and unpleasant buzzing noise alerts everyone in a 100m radius of your mistake.

The contrast between the tense, quiet focus of performing the "surgery" and the obnoxious, abrasive siren wail is enough to make a small child nigh on poop their pants. Especially sensitive children. I must have been a sensitive child...

Jokes aside, I found the game extremely unpleasant. The consequence of making a tiny "mistake" was HUGE! Not only did it scare the living shit out of me, but it also felt pretty humiliating. Especially as I was playing with people who had practiced a lot and seemed to never make mistakes. The loud buzzer seemed to announce (to me, anyway) - "HEY EVERYONE! CHECK IT OUT! ANDREW SUCKS AT THIS GAME! HE JUST KILLED THE PATIENT!"

For me, it was not only the buzzer-and-lights assault that was unpleasant. It was also that it was inevitably followed up

> *by the other kids laughing at how much I jumped when the buzzer sounded. Kids are rarely (if ever) coached on how to respond to other people's mistakes. And boy oh boy, do we ever make a cultural pastime of ridiculing each other!*

Now, you might say "Hey Andrew, you just need to toughen up, old boy! Who cares? It's just a game!" And I'd even be willing to credit that point - if indeed, this game was the only place that happened. But it's not - not by a long shot. I can remember offering answers out loud in class, only to be chastised for my mistakes by teachers, and mocked and humiliated by my fellow students. I can remember being punished by my parents for mistakes that I made as a child. I can recall with devastating clarity what our class did to the "weird kids" that didn't fit in so well. We tore them apart. It was savage.

When you take these things as a whole, you can see how they create a culture in which mistakes (or even *differences)* are to be deeply feared. For all but those with very thick skin, even the possibility of making a mistake or being different in front of others is terrifying. We know what happens to people who make mistakes - they are publicly crucified. Today more than ever, where mistakes can be blown way out of proportion, shared in outrage-inducing social media posts and receive millions of views, we can find ourselves trying to play it safe. After all, we don't want to be like *that guy* who said *that thing* and now the whole world treats him like a pariah!

Yes, mistakes can really suck, and yes, part of raising kids is to teach them not to mess up important things, but I believe we can do a much better job of it. In this chapter, I'd like to explain how vital mistakes can be, and how we can come to relate to them in better ways.

So how can Juggling Wisdom help us here?

Well, juggling requires learning. And learning is an area that produces a whole lot of anxiety for some of us. It's no wonder - we live in a very complex world. Every field of human endeavour is now light-years beyond what it was even a generation ago. Especially here in the Western world where our job prospects depend on a high degree of specialization, we need to be at the forefront of technology and be up to speed with state-of-the-art techniques. Suffice it to say, the necessity (and difficulty) of learning our way up to these extremely high standards is incredibly high. In fact, it's the highest that it's ever been in human history. So we ought to get our relationship to learning right!

I believe that we can use experiences in the juggling world as a light-hearted and safe way to explore our assorted relationships to learning. As I mentioned in part one, I believe that juggling is probably the most trivial and ridiculous pursuit there is. Well, maybe not the *most* trivial, but it's certainly up there. Somebody once described juggling to me as "doing the unnecessary, the hard way." And it's true! The act of juggling is totally unnecessary. And jugglers just *love* to come up with more and more obscure, difficult and convoluted ways of performing this totally unnecessary action.

But juggling is able to teach us *so much* about how we approach learning, what our deeply held beliefs and assumptions are, and provides us with a low-risk and fun way to go about diagnosing and changing our self-defeating tendencies.

There's probably a whole ton of definitions out there of the term "learning". I'll bet there's a bunch of very-qualified people who have written all sorts of theses, treatises, manuals, books, and studies of learning. And as a psychology graduate, I'm probably supposed to remember some of them. Well, the truth is, I actually believe that, in order for learning to be relevant, it has to *belong to us*. That is, *you* can't do my learning for me – I have to do it for myself. And in that spirit, I've created my own definition of learning, which may or may not overlap with other commonly accepted definitions. It is:

Learning is the process of coming to know, or being able to do something that you didn't know or couldn't do before.

Now that we're on the same page, let's break it down. There are two parts to this definition: the before and the after. Before, I *didn't* know/*couldn't* do. After, I *did* know/*could* do. Learning is what changes my state from the *before* category to the *after* category.

What people seem to forget is that, in order to learn, you need to begin in a state of *don't know/can't do*. You can't start out as an expert. You have to start out as a beginner, and move from low skill to high skill. And guess what beginners do – that's right! Make mistakes! Beginners make *all sorts* of mistakes because they don't know what the heck they're doing! Of course they don't! They're beginners! You probably wouldn't expect to be able to jump into a modern commercial jet and be able to fly it with no practice, would you? So why on earth would you expect to be able to perform the equally complex physical actions of juggling with no practice and succeed on the first try?!

It may sound ridiculous, but in my experience, many people *actually hold this expectation!* That they can try to juggle, and on the very first try, be able to juggle flawlessly without dropping. And when they *do* drop, they act as if it was a personal insult from the universe. Which then results in a feeling of outrage followed by quitting.

In defense of failure:

Most of us consider the pursuit of anything to have two outcomes: success and failure. Did you win or did you lose? Did you succeed or did you fail? However, I believe that failure IS the path to success. I've found that, with the occasional freak exception, success is only something that you get when you fail a whole bunch. I've noticed that successful people don't have talent or luck – they simply fail in almost all the ways it's possible to fail until the only path left is success. They've eaten dirt over and over again until they struck it rich. Successful people own each "failure" and use it to their advantage: it becomes an asset, as it has taught them something.

Sometimes "failure" is actually the best metric for success. Which sounds like nonsense. But consider the world of business, which mirrors juggling in that consistent failure is often the best indication that a business (or an aspiring juggler) will eventually succeed. If failure is the process of coming up against edges and learning the landscape, frequent failure gives you more information on which to base your next guesses. And, at their core, *all* of our decisions about future actions are really just guesses. We guess, and we hope, that if we say *this*, then we'll get *that*. That if we make this particular investment of time or energy, it'll pay off. All of our decisions are really just a series of educated guesses. We fool ourselves into thinking that our decisions are grounded in the certainty of our past knowledge and experience, but the truth is that nobody knows everything, and everybody is missing *something*.

We often think of endeavour as a path that ends in either success or failure. Either you win or you lose. I propose an alternative:

The path to success is paved with failures.

Each subsequent failure teaches us more about what success *isn't*. Failures are the paving stones along our journey to success. If we started with perfect knowledge of what success looks like and how to achieve it, we would be there already. It serves us well to get crystal clear on the true consequences of our "failures". Often we are terrified of them because we are feeding an untrue story of how the world will end when we fail.

There's a reason why we do this: we've made a cultural pastime out of ridiculing failures. We don't just laugh or criticise – we make people *feel bad* for their mistakes, even in times when they couldn't have known better. And this mockery has a cruel way of turning on the perpetrator: when we mock others for their failures, we are secretly telling ourselves that **we** are not allowed to fail. And by extension, that means we aren't allowed to try or to succeed.

The circus world has taught me that there's a better way – rather than ridiculing our failures, we should **celebrate** them.

The clown who takes a fall on purpose so that we can all laugh is a hero. They brave the world of failure and make it light so that we might take our own falls more lightly.

As long as we have the capacity to continue to endure these failures and make a commitment to learn from our mistakes and "fail forward", more failure means more learning, which means we're travelling faster on the path to success. And if we redefine our concept of "success" along the way, so much the better. These moments can present us with our greatest learnings, when we let go of definitions of success that don't serve us.

Success isn't about finding the right path on the first try. It's about eliminating wrong paths one by one until all that's left is the right one.

Back to our cultural trend toward mocking failure. For a number of years, anytime I would teach a group of kids to juggle, I would inevitably hear someone belt out "FAIL!", rather like the Operation buzzer, anytime someone made a mistake. Even if it was unrelated to juggling: someone might stumble on their way into the room and be greeted by a chorus of "FAIL!". It would drive me nuts to hear it every time. It builds exactly the wrong kind of environment to learn in. It's almost impossible not to shut down if even the most minor mistake is announced publicly and at full volume by a mocking peer. We need to stop mocking failure and start celebrating it.

I like to share the following thought experiment when I notice this happening in the group that I'm teaching:

That's it. I quit!

Think of when you were very very young, first learning to walk. Try to imagine your first attempts at walking. Do you think you got it right the first time and never fell? That you're the one human being ever who was able to master the skill without failure? Obviously not – you were a baby just like every other who was lucky enough to be born with legs and no idea how to use them.

So what happened instead? You fell. You got back up and tried it again and again until you got it. Maybe you hurt yourself and cried along the way, but hey – what baby in the world hasn't walked into a door or fallen on the hard floor? Those were the hard facts that taught you how to stand tall and why it's important.

Now imagine your first fall. Maybe you even bashed your head on a hard table edge or something. Yeah, it probably sucked either way. But imagine that, instead of getting over it and trying again, you'd taken that lesson and said to yourself "Nope! Can't do it! No way! That walking stuff... WAY too hard for me. I'm sitting this one out, guys. Y'all can just push me around in a wheelchair forever. I quit." Only you'd be a baby, so it'd sound more like "WAAAAAA!!!!"

Now fast forward to your current age. Imagine still being pushed around in a wheelchair because you made a single mistake and refused to learn to walk. You'd meet new people and they'd say to you "Hey, what happened to your legs? Did you break them?" "Oh, no. Just decided that they were too difficult to use." Only you probably wouldn't be able to say that, because if you'd decided to quit walking because it was too hard to learn, no way you would tackle the task of learning the English language (or whatever language you speak in)! English especially though...

Thankfully, some educators are realizing that the constant fear of mistakes is keeping students from trying. They have tried to address this by removing the possibility of failure. Unfortunately, this is even worse. In fact, I believe that the worst learning outcomes often come from an artificial separation of the participant from the possibility of failure. I was shocked when I learned that some schools have the policy that students are not allowed to fail tests or assignments. Which is to say that, even if they don't bother to complete and turn in an assignment, the teacher is not allowed to give them a mark of 0. I have heard of schools where the lowest mark teachers can give to students is 40%. And that's even if they never show up, and never turn in an assignment.

Imagine what that would do to a person's sense of consequences! I understand that a lot of students shut down because they are overwhelmed by the prospect of failure, but pretending that failure doesn't exist is NOT the way to deal with this! If we want students to avoid shutting down from fear of failure, *we need to reduce the unnecessary emotional cost of failure*, and make them more resilient. Failure doesn't have to mean embarrassment or weighty conclusions about one's self worth. In fact, failure can sometimes be the best part of an adventure.

As we explored in the last chapter, setting our definitions matters here: If I point my attention to one specific category, I might doubt the fact that I'm learning, even if I'm making enormous progress in a different, also-necessary dimension.

The importance of process vs. conclusion

Why do you do what you do? Is it to attain a particular outcome, or to participate in the process? Both process and conclusion are important, of course, but we must remember not to sell out one for the other. If we fixate on a "successful" outcome, it often means forsaking the opportunity to explore, make mistakes, and learn along the way. Likewise, if we focus too heavily on process, we may never even *get to* the conclusion!

Our culture's praise of success and mockery of failure has left us jaded about what I believe is the richest part of learning – the process. With more and more emphasis on the speed of information, efficiency, "productivity" (I put this in quotations because the mere act of producing has overshadowed our questioning of *what* we're producing, which is often trivial, wasteful, and completely misguided. I mean, come on! Dollar-store tools? They break before you even use them once!), we have lost sight of the value of the journey. The richest and most significant journeys are ones with ups and downs, challenges and triumphs, twists and turns.

If expertise was simply access to information, everyone with a smartphone in their pocket could be considered a pilot, surgeon, carpenter, fill-in-the-blank however you want. But true expertise, of course, isn't won simply by doing a google search on how to build a door frame, perform a surgery, or fly a plane. It is experience, it is repeated failure, it is a deep knowing that cannot be replaced by mere information. If a journey doesn't contain at least one mistake, what have you really learned?

I believe the truth is that we are actually very poor judges of what we should be learning. Life is so much bigger than we are that even our collective attempts to impart necessary skills on our youth (that is, our entire education system) is, in my opinion, questionably effective.

Pre-determined learning curriculums leave students with a wealth of skills that they'll never need, and a dearth of absolutely essential life skills. Calculus, trigonometry, literature (yes, YOU Shakespeare!), and many other subjects that most people can't make use of on a daily basis take the place that vitally relevant skills don't get – such as communication skills, financial literacy, nutrition and emotional regulation, just to name a few. I don't want this to turn into an education-bashing book, so I'll sum it up with one brief story and leave it at that:

Trust me - you'll need to know this someday!

I remember like it was yesterday, the dozens of arguments I had with teachers and other adults. Why do I need to know all this stuff? "Trust us, Andrew, you will someday!" was their inevitable answer. And I'm one of the lucky ones! Most academic stuff came really easily to me - I never had to try very hard to succeed in school.

And yet, I took offense at some of the things I was being asked to do. Quadratic equations, calculus, and trigonometry were at the forefront of my objections. I knew it. Everybody around me knew it – this stuff was garbage!

At least, to a teenager, it was. Sure, there are some people who really do need to know that stuff. But that's the key – **some** *people need it. Why couldn't they just learn it when it's time to do whatever-it-is-they-do-with-that-stuff? Why are they cramming this stuff down everyone's throat without discrimination?*

I felt like the adults knew just as well as we did that this stuff would be irrelevant to most of us, but maybe it felt too much like it was their job to teach us to be able to admit it. And so they soldiered on, steamrolling everyone with these lessons. I learned calculus, trigonometry, and all the etceteras., as it was made clear to me that I didn't have any choice in the matter.

Now, 15 years later, I finally have occasion to use the skills. Trigonometry, specifically. And before you jump up and down and shout "See! I knew it! All of us responsible adults **knew** *you'd need it!", wait until I finish. See, a friend of mine learned of my interest in woodworking, and had a project in mind. Someone had made her a loft bed, but left out the ladder. She had to use an ugly aluminum Canadian Tire ladder that stretched all the way up to the ceiling to get into her nice wooden loft bed. So she asked me to make her a ladder. Great!*

After taking measurements of the height, length, and width of the space, I can go buy the lumber. Now I need to cut the wood to the proper angles to butt up flat against both the bed and the floor. I try to dredge the formulas out of my cluttered head – SOH CAH TOA, right? I remember sine, cosine, and tangent, but I don't remember what to do with them. I spend a bit of time trying to figure it out, but then realize: Hey – I bet Google can solve this problem for me in about 0.14873 seconds.

I punch the numbers in, and sure enough, Google solves the problem for me in precisely 0.14873 seconds, giving me all of the relevant angles. I went on to make the ladder and all was well.

So – is this a story of me "cheating"? That I "should have" calculated it myself rather than rely on Google? Could I have done the calculations manually? Well, no – sine, cosine, and tangent were all functions that could only be performed by a calculator, as far as we were taught.

No, I think this is a story of how somebody (or several somebodies, who wrote the math curriculum) was **convinced** that they knew what I needed to learn in order to be successful. And they were wrong. By a long shot. Take a moment to think about how many of our collective resources went into (and STILL go into) the indiscriminate teaching of non-useful subjects to our youth. Curriculum design, writing textbooks, classroom space, training teachers to teach it, software and other tools to help teach it, even the social resources that are expended - think of how much damage it does to the confidence our youth have in our judgement when we FORCE them through these irrelevant lessons.

Think also about how many young people come out of these lessons with the idea that they're not good learners because they don't get it...

And I believe that the scale of these consequences is MASSIVE. Turning young adults off of learning has *decades or generations* of repercussions. Is it really worth all that to insist that students learn this or that specific thing? Doesn't anyone care that young people have virtually no agency to determine the path of their own education?

So what's my point? Is it that we shouldn't be teaching math to kids? No, that's not what I'm saying. What I'm saying is that we're too damn sure of ourselves and our ability to predict the future. Our confidence in our predictions leads us to overcommit our resources in losing bets. We are oh-so-sure that we know what's relevant and irrelevant; we seem to have no humility at all, and so we leave no room for doubt. History has shown us over and over and over again just how prone we are to cultural biases and blind spots, and that we sometimes miss really big things that are right in front of us.

I think this is one of those big things right in front of us. We approach education as "Here's what you're going to do, kid. Now get to it!" We approach things as if the child or teen has nothing useful to tell us about their own educational preferences or needs. And even if they can summon the courage to ask, they're not always going to get the accommodation or the agency that they want. Most educational environments are pretty low-trust - we start with the assumption that kids are so irresponsible that they need to be constantly corralled and forced to learn, and not only that, but we adults need to make all of the decisions of what they learn and when. This may not seem like a big deal, but think about all of the zest for learning that gets lost when someone is continually railroaded into a path that doesn't line up with their interests.

Growing up with your sense of agency in your own learning constantly being undermined is profoundly disempowering.

     I also want to clarify and say that I don't think I am much better (than our education system) at planning for and learning the skills that I'll need in the future. If I had that kind of foresight, I'd be playing the lottery instead of writing this book! I didn't realize that acrobatics, juggling, and comedy skills were going to be so essential to me. If I had, I would have started learning them earlier in my life.

     At best, I have a mediocre sense of what I need to know *now*. I continue to struggle daily as a husband and father with conflicts and hardships that come from not having all the skills I need to navigate these roles. And even though I try to be open to the learnings that come up, it's seriously challenging. If you ask me today what skills I'm going to have to use tomorrow when I am homeschooling my son for the day, I probably couldn't tell you.

One thing that I *do* know for sure is that I am more likely to be adequately prepared for tomorrow's challenges if I give up the arrogant view that I know what I should be learning. I have found that there is great wisdom in being open to the lessons that life gives, even if they don't fit my idea of what I "should" be learning.

     Life is a voyage into the unknown. You have an entirely new landscape to explore and understand every time you do anything new. The only way to really know the landscape is to explore it. And that means coming up against edges. This can sometimes be an unpleasant experience. It's trying something and having it not work out the way you'd expected.

But when we do this, it provides us with valuable information with which to guide our next action. If we don't receive that feedback, our next action will be made in ignorance of the thing we might otherwise have learned.

I'll share a story of a time when I decided to challenge myself to wear a blindfold for 10 days and nights, and be effectively blind for that time period. It was back when I was young enough that I didn't have any serious responsibilities and had the luxury of doing so with support from others.

My experience of blindness

When I grew up, I had the privilege of wrestling at the W. Ross MacDonald School for the Blind. From grades 5-12, I went to the blind school to practice wrestling skills with a team of both blind and sighted wrestlers. Due to the generosity of Wayne Gretzky, who had donated some very expensive, high-quality wrestling mats, and the incredible coaching of two men – Mr. Zinger (who is an Olympic-level referee and very well-respected in the world of wrestling), and John Howe, incredible teacher and leader, and principal of the school, we had a great team. This meant that I had the chance to become friends with, wrestle against, and guide several blind athletes, a responsibility that I took very seriously.

I recall that, in order to volunteer at the school (something that I never formally did), one had to wear a blindfold for some period (between one and three days, I think). I thought that this was a great idea, but at the time, no one ever suggested that I try it, and I had plenty on my plate already.

Anyway, I came back to it years later and decided to try it, and up the ante by doing it for a full 10 days. I wanted to go about my life as normally as possible, including visits to the University of Guelph Juggling Club, and riding my unicycle.

I remember trying to ride my unicycle blind, but it was absolutely terrifying. Every moment, I felt convinced that I was going to crash into something. I had somebody who I trusted guiding me verbally. I decided to try it just outside my house – at the time I was living in a townhouse complex with winding laneways and minor speed bumps. Picture a pac-man

> *level. As I rode, I didn't bump into anything, but felt increasing anxiety anyway. I found myself wishing that I **could** bump into a wall so that I would know where I was.*
>
> *Being out in the open when you're blind is terrifying – not only do you feel like you could be anywhere, you also don't even know which direction you're oriented in!*
>
> *One detail that I took out of the experience was that it was impossible to navigate a space on my own without access to a wall. I learned that it was often worth the crash into the wall just to know where I was. Even in my very small kitchen – if I ventured from the safety of the fridge into the enormous unknown gulf of 5-6 steps to the sink, I'd often miss my target. With this in mind, I decided that the stove was much to risky to try...*

Walls are great when you're blind because they let you know where you are, and give you some clue as to how to get to your destination, or even just how to navigate the space. I think that this is true of all edges – they give us information that we can use to make better decisions. The more we know about the edges, the shape of the landscape, the better informed we are when we decide how to interact with it. Whether it's an opportunity, a physical space, an idea, or a relationship, we will be able to make better decisions when we know the shape of what we're dealing with.

Making a mistake is like bumping into the edge of something. It shows you the limits. Mistakes tell you where a thing ends. And not all mistakes are created equal – bumping into a wall is not the same thing as bumping into a transport truck on the highway. Yes, some mistakes will kill you. But sometimes we go around treating *all* mistakes as if they'll kill us.

Maybe we feel like they will – maybe we're holding onto an idea of who we are that is fragile, and making a mistake might break that image. Whether you have an over-inflated or a diminished sense of self, this can be true.

I believe that it is the mistakes that most threaten our sense of self that we are most averse to making.

If life is a big process of navigating the unknown, why aren't we more interested in what that landscape *actually* looks like? Shouldn't we *want* to know where the edges are? This idea feels self-evident when you really think about it. There are many great models of this principle, among them two of my favourite authors – Malcolm Gladwell (whose father taught him how much there is to learn when you abandon your intellectual insecurities and aren't afraid to look like a fool by not knowing), and Ray Dalio (who has made it his life's work to systematically explore all of the errors in his thinking in an effort to develop an ever-increasingly robust model of the world.) Both of these authors delight in finding out that they're wrong – because it means that they are one step closer to being right!

So what's the story we're telling about ourselves that's so threatened by our mistakes?

Well, frankly, I think it's a story being told by our egos. And before you go burning our egos at the stake, understand that this, too, serves an important function in our lives. Ego (in this case, our attachment to the notion that we are right) gives us the confidence to act. The certainty that our ego gives us allows us to make decisions quickly without having to demolish and rebuild our framework with every decision we're faced with. It says "Door A is the right door, I'm sure of it – that's where we're going".

Without this voice, we might get lost in the confusion of the endless alternatives in the world. Ego allows us to make decisions quickly by closing off all of the alternative possibilities so that we don't deliberate endlessly over each choice. Where this becomes a problem is with decisions that shouldn't be made so quickly (or when we're just plain wrong).

Another difficulty our egos lead us into is having to prove others wrong in order to continue to feel right. Our egos (especially when we feed them too much), try to have us look like the best person in the room so that our frameworks will be taken as superior to all others in the room.

Our egos are fed in times when we are correct or look good in front of a group, and we come to understand that this is who we are. Similarly, when we make mistakes, it gives us the overwhelming desire to explain ourselves and justify our mistake.

Our egos have us believing that we **are** our success or failure. We *want* to be successful, of course! It feels great! When everyone looks at us and praises us for that thing we did, we want to hang that trophy on our wall and believe that **it is who we are.** But when we fail, we want to distance our sense of selves from what just happened: "Oh, it's not my fault – you're the one who told me the wrong thing!".

This constant waltz toward success and away from failure that our egos take us on can often make us dizzy and confused, unable to see reality properly. It stops us from seeing that we are so much more than our successes or failures.

If we buy into the stories of our egos, we avoid mistakes because we believe that these failures define who we are, not what we've done.

This tendency of our egos is particularly deadly when combined with our often-inaccurate estimations of our own skills or ability to learn. When it comes to physical skills, I have found that an alarming number of people have very poor opinions of themselves. These poor estimates of skill and the certainty with which we hold them sets the stage for the final blow – that if we fail, others will think less of us (which they surely must do, because **we** look at the world through that lens!)

If we believe our worth in this world is tied to looking good to others and to ourselves, we won't allow ourselves to take the risk of making mistakes. And my experience is that we're often totally unaware of doing this, and we only catch up with the consequences several steps down the road.

I have found that there are two ways of dealing with this:

- Separate our sense of self from our performance

- Reduce the negative consequences* of our mistakes where possible

---

*It's very important that we only reduce the negative consequences as opposed to all consequences – remember that mistakes are absolutely vital to learning. If we insulate ourselves from all consequences, we can't learn!

- **Separating our sense of self from our performance**

Gosh, I can't believe that I've put this into a bullet point. It's actually a life pursuit, and takes a lifetime to practice. This point truly deserves a book of its own, but I'll do my best to stay on topic here!

First I'd like to point you in the direction of an author whose work is specifically centred on this subject, and he says it much better than I can. Michael Singer, who wrote The Untethered Soul and The Surrender Experiment, explains that our attachment to our ideas of who we are gets in the way of all sorts of things. In short, we can't truly be *in* reality while we're in our heads, mulling over and over our stories of how things "should" be.

We think we know how everything is supposed to be, despite the universe being far bigger and far older than we can even conceive. As tiny, brief specks in the span of the universe, we are almost entirely inconsequential in the grand scheme of things, yet we walk around as if we ought to be the one with the conductor's baton, orchestrating everything around us. And rather than living in the real world, most of us are living in "the world as it relates to me and my interests". And while we are participating in this worldview, we are taking all of the resources in our brains away from being present with what is.

It's the basic concept of mindfulness and presence, taught in Buddhism and meditation – get out of your head and get into reality. Your head tells you strange and off-putting things all the time (such as "No, I can't drop the ball in front of Charlotte – she'll think less of me!" or "I can't admit that mistake to my wife – she'll never trust me again!"), but juggling balls will never criticize you for dropping them!

The real world doesn't care one way or another whether you succeed on your first or seventh try, and if you are practiced at sitting in the real world (as opposed to buying into the silly-ass stories bouncing around in your head), you'll have the freedom to try and fail and learn without all the guilt and heaviness hanging over you.

Now, you may not feel like I'm describing you with the above, but I would invite you to ask yourself if that really **is** true, or if that's just what your ego is telling you.

Here's a little experiment for you:

Play dumb

*Pick a subject or an activity that you know a lot about. More than your average person. Then ask someone to explain it to you as if you don't know anything. When they tell you about it, notice the urge to correct them on points where they differ from how you would have explained it. I'm guessing that you'll notice yourself (at least in your head) pointing out their errors, or supplementing the information somehow. You might even feel the urge to explain the experiment to them afterward, just so that it's clear that you **are,** in fact, an expert on the subject.*

How else could you explain these thoughts and urges except that they are born from a desire to prove yourself? And don't try to pretend that you're doing them a favour by correcting their explanation! Come on, ego, we can see right through you! In the end, you don't correct people because you care at all about them getting it right, you do it because it makes you right. That's your ego, and it's ok that you have one – it's part of what makes you human. Just acknowledge it, give it a hug, and take your executive functions back!

But what if I'm doing something where making mistakes is really really bad?

Alright, say you're a surgeon, or a pilot or a military general, and lives depend on your getting it right. I would argue that it is *especially* important for you to have a good relationship with your mistakes. For you, as with all human beings, it's not a question of *if* you make mistakes, it's a question of when. If mistakes are a given (and I believe that they are), then it makes sense to develop a good way to relate to them.

Let me put it to you this way – if *you* were relying on a surgeon, pilot, or military general, would you want them to:

- **A** – Believe that they shouldn't make mistakes, and when they do, either deny they made them or get crushed with guilt?
  OR
- **B** – Admit the mistake and learn from it to reduce the likelihood of further mistakes?

Personally, I'd choose B. And I understand how mistakes can feel so heavy, so abhorrent that it can feel impossible to even look at them. As a parent, I'm familiar with the tension that comes from the responsibility to not mess up my kid by making mistakes. It definitely feels heavy at times. I also work as a professional speaker at large events with hundreds or thousands of guests, where the pressure is also great to not make mistakes. Sure, they're not life-or-death mistakes, but I can definitely identify with the pressure to get it right.

Remember that burnout is a real thing - I believe that a huge component of burnout in high-pressure jobs comes from not knowing how to relate to the high-impact mistakes that are inevitable over time.

So if you're in a situation where the stakes are high, you can recognize that this might be the time to prioritize results over making mistakes & learning – but it's important to also recognize that your learning needs to happen somewhere.

You can set up scenarios with lower stakes if you want to learn, which brings me to the next strategy:

• **Reduce the negative consequences of failure**

Reducing negative consequences of failure can happen in one of two ways: by changing the way that we relate to the consequences, and by changing the consequences themselves. That is, we can change the *outcome* (outside of ourselves) from our mistakes, or we can change our feelings (inside of ourselves) about those mistakes. I believe that both are very important to consider if we want to have a more optimized relationship to risk-taking.

An example of the first category (changing consequences) would be to practice in a low-risk environment that is designed for learning. In the Operation game, it would mean taking the damn battery out of the game so it can't give you a heart-attack! Think pilot simulator games, a driving obstacle course, or rehearsing a speech to your couch rather than a full audience. If you stutter in your introduction, your couch isn't going to think less of you!

This approach is especially important for learning truly high-risk skills (that is, where the external risk is high). It is incredibly useful to be able to learn and make mistakes in a safe context where lives aren't on the line, and helps us to establish a calm baseline of emotion during the brain-stretching process of learning.

It makes sense, doesn't it, to take the external risks of failure out for learning? If you're lucky enough to have access to gym mats and a spotter, it makes learning a backflip a lot easier. If there is external pressure to get it right, this approach facilitates learning by removing that pressure. The examples so far have been pretty straightforward, so let's look at a few that are more nuanced.

Let's say that you need to have a difficult conversation with your boss about your working conditions, your pay, or your experience of a co-worker. Perhaps it feels like there are high external stakes to this conversation – if you are not successful in persuading your boss to see your point of view, it might mean that you have to continue working in unsafe conditions, or you will continue to resent your work because you feel that you are underpaid, or that you have to endure further harassment from your co-worker. It is not uncommon to feel so much pressure attached to this interaction that we put it off and put it off out of fear of failure, and never actually have that necessary conversation.

I could propose having a "practice conversation" with a friend or someone else you trust, but I doubt that you'd find the advice to be very useful. This is because I don't think that we make most of our risk decisions based on external risks (even if those are the factors we tend to cite). Almost no one *reads statistics* on actual risk levels when they choose not to do something – if they did, people would sooner steer clear of badminton than rock climbing. There is statistically a much greater chance of getting injured playing badminton than rock climbing - look it up if you don't believe me!

The reason that I believe that we don't make our risk decisions based on data is that we most often make our decisions from an almost complete absence of data. When's the last time that you looked up evidence for the safety of something before deciding whether you should do it? In my experience, I've addressed people's objections, as one by one they continue to create new objections on the spot as to why they can't do something such as learning to juggle, do a handstand, or unicycle. It feels clear to me that these are emotion-based objections rather than factual, data-driven objections.

So if we don't make risk decisions based on evidence around external risks, what *do* we use to make our decisions? I believe that we only ever consider internal factors, even though we say otherwise.

We come up with internal fantasies of how external risks might play out, and then make our decisions based on those fantasies.

The ease with which we can, and regularly do, imagine our failures and their consequences makes them feel more likely. I can imagine just how bad that broken leg would be, so even if it's only a one-in-a-million chance, I almost consider it to have already happened. Because it did! In my imagination, anyway. But then my nervous system reacts and now I'm making the decision from the basis of my biological response to it. Which is a very macro-wise point of view - it's the instinct that kept our ancestors alive long enough to beget us! The problem is, it's not so appropriate on the micro scale of our lives and the thing that's in front of us.

Even abstract social risks and emotional risks are calculated this way. It's dangerous to disagree, to stand out, to show ineptitude. Our same wise ancestors would have cast us out for such things as being different or inept. We kept our share of resources in the herd by blending in. Whether that's an accurate story or not seems not to matter - when we examine our feelings toward these types of risk, we *know well* how viscerally terrifying it can be to break those social conventions, to defy common "prudent" behaviour.

Don't believe me? Give this a try:

Just make it up!

Grab some makeup from someone you know. I'm not talking about foundation and blush - I'm talking about face-paint in vivid colours. You can even promise them part of the fun that ensues - it'll be worth it. That is, if you can actually bring yourself to do it. This is a very difficult experiment.

Most people absolutely could not bring themselves to do it. With that makeup, I want you to draw on your own face the way a small child would. In fact, if you have access to a small child, I'd bet they'd be thrilled if you lent them your face as a canvas!

With your beautiful new face, go out into a public spot where everyone gets to admire the artwork. Even better, go about your normal business - grocery shopping, walk around the block, hang out with friends.

I know that you're not going to do this (all but a very few of you, anyway), but it doesn't matter. You'll nevertheless have imagined it with enough detail as to reveal your mortification at the possibility.

Now I'll admit here that in my first attempts at doing stage makeup on myself for circus shows, I wasn't able to make it look much better than what a small child would draw. And I will admit that it felt embarrassing to make myself get out on stage under the bright lights with makeup that I wasn't great at, but then I actually realized that the stage was something to lean on, so to speak. Even though I was socialized for my whole life in no uncertain terms that men absolutely MAY NOT wear makeup, I could justify this by being on stage, where it is expected.

What turned out to be the actual hard part was wearing that same terrible makeup while going shopping because there's only 20 minutes between shows, and I've gotta get food, shove it down my gullet and be ready to get back on stage in 20 minutes. And that certainly left no time for either makeup removal or re-application!

To tell the truth, if I didn't have that **necessity to do it** *the first time, I don't know that I would have gotten over the fear of doing it. But after I did, it didn't become a matter of necessity, it became a matter of laziness. I wouldn't bother taking off my makeup even if we weren't doing a show until next week!*

Well, maybe not quite... But hey, there were times when I stopped even noticing. Being able to appear wacky or weird or judge-able in front of others became just second nature to me. And that meant that I had so many more of my mental resources for the other things I was doing. Like trying to be able to step into the circus ring without nearly having a heart-attack each and every time.

When it comes to social risk aversion, our imaginations have a lot to say. We are so capable of weaving a whole story based on just a shred of truth, and we often get taken unknowingly on that ride. Which isn't a problem in itself – it only becomes a problem when we treat our imagined story as an accurate account of what's going to happen in reality. Enormous branches of possibility get lost to us because our imaginations love feeding us stories of risk. And those stories are so emotionally engaging that we are too horrified to apply logic, reason, or analysis before we make our decision to avoid something.

Back to that conversation with your boss. Now, my skills as a juggler don't exactly qualify me to coach you through that conversation, but I can certainly discuss ways of reducing the negative consequences. First, we can address your objectives. If you set out with the objective of *convincing* your boss to take your viewpoint and make the decision you would make, the odds of getting an unfavourable outcome increase.

This is because you do not control the thoughts, priorities, or decision-making framework of your boss (even if you think you ought to). You are essentially throwing something really important out into the wind and hoping that it'll blow in the direction you want it to.

If you define success as having your boss agree with you, you are making your window of success much smaller and harder to hit. Even if your issue is very important (I would say *especially* if your issue is very important), your conversation will have a much better chance to address your issues if you adopt a different definition of success.

If you approach the conversation instead as a chance to clearly articulate some information that is relevant to your experience, then simply by having the conversation, you are successful.

At the end of the day, even the most persuasive argument is unlikely to change your boss's decision-making framework – that never really *was* an option to begin with. Wouldn't you rather succeed in the ways you can – such as by clearly articulating your experience and some suggested courses of action? It may sound counterintuitive to reduce external consequences of failure by changing your approach internally, but you can see how they're connected – if you make *showing up and giving your best effort* your definition of success, it will save you from a whole world of unnecessary fallout. You don't have to believe that your efforts were in vain, you don't have to second-guess yourself or sabotage further efforts toward speaking up for yourself.

We can apply the same approach to any number of social risks that we find ourselves hesitant to make – the same principle applies. As we discussed at length in the previous chapter, *how we set our definitions really matters.*

Most of the "negative consequences" that we fear so deeply are actually nothing more than poorly chosen definitions.

While it can be easy to identify the external risks of our actions, the inner risks aren't so easily identified or understood. If I'm learning to juggle chainsaws, the dangers of catching the wrong end are so much more obvious and easily avoided – just don't turn the dang things on! But if I have an inner resistance to learning to juggle in front of others, it takes a whole lot more looking to identify the reason behind it (and furthermore, what to do about it!). Self-discovery can be painful, and requires real courage. Even apart from the embarrassment of dropping a ball in front of others, there's the difficulty of having to admit to yourself that you've got something weird going on in your head if juggling feels that scary.

If reducing external risks means setting up a safe external environment (using simulations, safety equipment, and accurate goal-setting), reducing internal risks means setting up a safe internal environment. This is much more easily said than done – you can't exactly go out to the hardware store and buy safety goggles for your mind! What you *can* do is work on separating your sense of self from the outcome of your endeavours. You can practice compassion with yourself and think logically about the necessity of mistakes in learning. You can also take those mistakes and turn them into a source of joy.

Celebrate the Flop!

The Jester of the Ski Hill

I'm flying downwards at some preposterous speed. Cold air whips across my face, numbing my skin. My heart is pounding in exhilaration. Snow is spraying up in all directions as my skis carve across the hill. This is my first time skiing on a real hill (as opposed to the training hill), and I'm having a blast. I had learned how to turn back and forth in a controlled journey down the hill and am confidently whipping back and forth, with a feeling that I'm on top of the world.

But at some point, the speed changes from exhilarating to terrifying. Maybe it's when I realize that I'm no longer in control. Somewhere along the way, my confident back-and-forth carving turns into a barely perceptible side-to-side sway. My ankles no longer feel like they're up to the challenge of slowing me down.

"Oh god! Ohgodohgodohgod!" I yell as my speed continues to pick up until I'm sailing, impossibly fast and out of control in a straight line down the hill. My zipper with ski tag attached is whipping me repeatedly in the face, chastising me for my overconfidence. My mom warned me about this! And of course I ignored her, rolling my eyes in typical 12-year-old fashion. It was our school's skiing trip - what was I supposed to do? Not go just because my mom was worried about me?

None of this matters, of course, as I'm convinced that these are the last moments of my life. A perfect time to take up religion again, I decide as I pray for my life. I'll never roll my eyes at my mom again, I swear!

One last attempt to reduce speed by turning my skis into that wedge-shape that's supposed to slow you down and stop you (it worked on the bunny hill – why not here!), somehow sends me flying end-over-end in a spectacular display of flailing limbs. Crashing awkwardly face-first into the snow, I eventually skid to a stop. To make it worse, I'm directly under the ski lift and everybody travelling up has seen my embarrassing crash. As I check my limbs to see if I still have feeling or if I have, in fact, broken my spine, neck, and all other bones in my body, I hear something from above me.

"Woooo! Yeah! Nice one! Hey dude, are you ok? That was a hell of a wipeout!" The trio above me are hooting and hollering at my unintentional acrobatics. Maybe it was the thrill I felt at still being alive, with all my limbs working and no apparent injury, or maybe it was the enthusiasm of the group above me, but I felt great! In fact, I burst out laughing and decided to do it again. My spectacular failure, having been celebrated by random skiers on the lift above me, was more fun than I'd had in a long time.

Hiking carefully around the hill to collect my strewn-about skis, I descended the remaining portion of the hill and got back on the lift, planning my next crash. I spent the whole day in spectacular wipeouts for the lift riders, an impromptu jester of the ski hill. And I had a great time!

Each round I would deliberately go too fast, and eat snow in the most outrageous crashes, and each time I was applauded by those riding the ski lift. I imagined that even those who did not applaud may have taken something from it – "I may not be great at skiing, but at least I'm not THAT guy!"

Leaving the hill at the end of the day, I had my share of well-earned bruises, but my spirits were high and I like to imagine that I raised others spirits as well.

I didn't realize it at the time, but what I was doing was clowning. Clowns deliberately fail at simple and obvious things, and we can all identify with that. Like searching frantically for our keys for ten minutes before realizing that they've been in our hands the whole time. Or thinking that it's a push-door when really it's a pull-door, and walking straight into it. These things can be embarrassing and we tend to store them up as tension. Clowns let us relive our mistakes, our "flops", in a safe environment where we can all have a good laugh at it and release that tension. We don't feel bad for the clown because they make their problems so obvious that they don't seem real. We know that they're doing it for us as a gift.

What about more serious mistakes? Like with actual doctors as opposed to kids crowded around a silly old board game? Shouldn't we avoid those at all costs, even if it means higher stress for people with responsibilities? Isn't it irresponsible to suggest that life-and-death mistakes should be treated the same way as mistakes in a game? Well, yes, it is. Some mistakes are serious and need to be treated with an appropriate sense of gravity. Nevertheless, we are humans and not a single one of us is infallible.

Mistakes will happen, no matter how much pressure we put on ourselves to get it right. What matters here is that we don't let our mistakes crush us completely and stop us from acting.

After all, if we've made a mistake, there is an unspoken burden on us to make it right. Even if our mistake is irreversible, we are still responsible for making sure that we (and others) don't make that same mistake again. However, if we're crushed with guilt, we lose our capacity to do this. The most important thing about this is feeling like mistakes don't have to be so damn heavy. When the Operation dude buzzes at us for failing to take the "funny bone" out of his elbow, laugh at him! (Not in real life though - doctors, take good care of our funny bones please and thanks!) Most mistakes that we make have no inherent cost to them other than inconvenience and embarrassment. Both of which are pretty trivial when we step back and look at them in perspective.

In fact, I've found that mistakes can be gifts, to remind us to take a better perspective and be able to laugh at ourselves. And if we can laugh in celebration rather than mockery, it gives others permission to do the same.

When our mistakes don't cost so much, we are more free to make them, and that means we are more free to learn.

I would love to see people start to re-brand failures or mistakes as gifts. Often when I teach a juggling workshop, I'll coach my students to respond to a drop by throwing their arms wide and presenting themselves with a big "Ta-da!" When I do this, I get the feedback that it makes the whole activity more enjoyable, much more like play than like work.

Own your mistakes.

I consider my bruises to be badges of honour. They are a testament to the strength of my spirit and what I have endured. In fact, I actually find activities and tasks much more rewarding when I have had to pay a high cost to participate. It means that, even though it was difficult, even though I got hurt, here I am at the end of the day, still standing. We've all heard the maxim "What doesn't kill us makes us stronger." I don't necessarily agree with this – sometimes our mistakes leave us with scars that impede our ability to perform in the future. I could lose my hand in a silly chainsaw-juggling accident and, while it may not kill me, I'm certainly not as strong as I'd be with both my hands still attached!

Rather than getting stuck on the wording though, I'd like to explore what's behind that saying. Mistakes, bruises, and bad experiences can teach us (if we let them) that, even when bad things happen, even when things don't go according to our expectations, we're still alive. That we made it through, even when we may have thought it impossible. So the next time we're afraid of a bad outcome, we can draw back on our experiences from the past and know that we've made it through tough times before.

There's a great Stephen Covey (7 Habits of Highly Effective People) quote: "Private victories precede public victories." I believe wholeheartedly in this. Every major victory that I have had in my life has only come about as a result of the struggles that came before it. Standing in front of an audience of thousands, performing extremely difficult acrobatic or juggling feats, when my anxiety levels are through the roof is not an easy task.

Most people wouldn't be able to do it, but that's only because most people haven't been through what I have been through. Just as I wouldn't be able to make the all-too-real life and death decisions that many people have to make every day - I haven't gone through what *they* had to go through to be able to make those decisions.

Every struggle, every bruise, every failure that I've experienced in the past, I bring with me onto the stage. I use them to keep me humble, to remind me that I'm only human. I also use them to remind me of how strong I am, of how much I can take and keep on ticking. The unshakeable confidence required to be out there "in the arena" comes from the knowledge that even if I fail, make a mistake, or screw up in some way, I'll still be there at the end of the day, and at least I had the guts to try. To go out there and do something that's meaningful to me, something that I believe the world needs.

We all have this ability, to endure things like embarrassment when necessary - I'll bet you can think of at least one intensely emotional experience that you had no idea how you were going to make it through at the time. However, your reading this book is proof that you made it through anyhow. You're stronger than you think.

When we can rally the strength to do it, owning our mistakes proves that we have earned the learning. When we leave our mistakes behind by denying that we made them, we are denying ourselves the learning that *we already suffered to gain!*

If we don't own our mistakes, we don't own our learning.

I think that most of us have had experience at one time or another with someone (often an authority figure. Perhaps a president?) who won't own up to their mistakes. What does that look like from the outside? Not so great, eh? Let me tell you a quick story of a time when I didn't own up to my mistake, that I still feel pretty embarrassed about. For some context, at the time, I ran a circus school, in which I taught circus skills to youth and adults.

Stood up

I got a call about a gig, and I was pretty excited. I hadn't been working for very long as a freelance artist, so gigs were still relatively rare and certainly exciting. This particular request was for a performance at a nursing home. They were having a big circus-themed event, and the organizer sought me out specifically as the headliner for the event. The residents of this nursing home had a day of festivities, which included carnival games, popcorn, cotton candy, and my job was to be the entertainment for the dinner. I had a whole 45-minute solo show which included juggling, acrobatics, unicycling, and comedy, and I was excited to perform.

Weeks passed as I prepared for it. I did so much work on my performance, actually, that I lost my normal anxiety around it. I took it as a sign that I was being pretty responsible. Hey, I'm finally getting the hang of being a professional!

One night, after I'm finished coaching at the circus school and I'm checking my phone, I get a strange feeling. I have 5 new messages. Confused as to who wanted to get a hold of me so badly, I start playing back the messages. My heart sinks.

"Hey Andrew, it's Kelly. I just wanted to let you know that you can park in the lot beside the side doors, and bring your things in through the red doors near the back. Let me know when you arrive and I'll come out and meet you. We're all really excited to see your performance tonight!"

You can guess how the next 4 messages played out. I forced myself to listen through each of them as Kelly went through the emotional range between confusion, worry, irritation, outrage, and finally giving up. I felt awful. I couldn't believe how bad a mistake I'd made. I let down an audience of hundreds, an organizer that had done a lot of work to arrange the event, and even myself. How could I have let this happen?

I was absolutely **crushed** with guilt. It felt fully impossible to face the consequences of this. To admit to Kelly and all the residents of the nursing home that I'd let them down for the simple reason that I forgot to check my calendar and thus forgot the performance. I beat myself up for the next 30 minutes before I was finally able to pick up the phone and call Kelly back. I owed her at least that much.

I'm embarrassed by this whole story, but particularly about what happened next. When I called Kelly back, I lied to her about why I had missed the show. I told her that there was an emergency and I had to take my brother to the hospital and forgot my phone. I just didn't feel like I could own my mistake because it seemed too horrible to admit to it. And when I responded by lying about it rather than owning up to it, I made an even greater mistake.

In the end, I'll bet that Kelly didn't even buy my BS brother-in-the-hospital story anyway. So now I was an asshole for two reasons rather than one. An innocent (even if crushingly embarrassing) scheduling mistake is one thing, but deliberately and blatantly lying about it to avoid responsibility probably made me look 10 times worse.

I offered to perform a make-up show some other time, and offer a few extra services to make up for the mistake, but she never took me up on it. I'm not surprised – I broke her trust

> *pretty badly. The stood-up audience was so disappointed, and I have to carry this story with me now. I feel that I owe it to them to admit my mistake, and use the experience to grow and do a better job next time. I also owe it to my **future** audiences to admit my mistake, get a better scheduling system, and not repeat my error. Most importantly, I owe it to myself to be honest and not lie again in a childish attempt to avoid blame.*

Mistakes are like a gas leak – sometimes they stink real bad, but they tell you something you REALLY need to know. Our biggest challenge is to be mature and courageous enough to face up to them and learn our lessons.

What it looks like

Even after all this talk of making mistakes, it can be challenging to know what to do in the moment. We've messed up, and there we are with our big bad embarrassing mistake dangling out in the open where everyone can see, and maybe we're wishing that we could turn invisible, turn back time, or use a miracle to turn the mistake into something else.

All of this philosophy means nothing unless we can have the courage to put it into practice in those hard moments.

First, I'd like to acknowledge that, even though I'm writing a book on this, I don't always succeed in practicing my advice. But when I do make a point to own my mistakes, I have found that it is actually the quickest and least hasslesome exit from the situation. It gets to the point right away so that things can be resolved more easily. It avoids drawing the issue out into he-said-she-said nonsense that feels crummy and gets us nowhere.

What it looks like, first and foremost, is acknowledging and accepting that my mistake happened. Again, this can feel tough because it brings with it the implication that **I** was wrong (rather than *my choice* being wrong). True admission of a mistake doesn't try to justify, excuse, or diminish what happened. I can do this through simple and factual statements such as: "I dropped the ball", "I forgot to pick you up from the airport", "I made an error in judgement", or "It turns out that was the wrong thing to do."

Even if it hurts, I have to acknowledge the truth of these statements. If I forgot to pick up my friend from the airport, I forgot to pick up my friend from the airport. This statement is true regardless of how I or my friend may feel about it. My feelings are an entirely separate issue.

When we start with this acknowledgement, it avoids a whole world of unnecessary finger-pointing, dissecting, and unpleasant rehashing of the incident. No one likes that – it's unproductive and it feels shitty. But with the truth right out there on the table, all parties can move on to the next step, which is dealing with the feelings and other consequences around it.

The next step is the hard one. In fact, the only reason the first step is hard is because it leads to the second step, which is acknowledging the impact that the mistake has had. As we explored, the actual impact is often made up anyway (usually it boils down to feelings – I feel uncomfortable because I dropped a ball in front of people. You feel irritated because I left you stranded at the airport. I feel disappointed because you forgot my birthday).

Regardless of whether the consequences are in the physical world or the ethereal world of feelings and relationships, we still need to acknowledge and deal with them as well. Successful practitioners of this skill don't try to diminish, negate, or deny the consequences of what they've done. They have the courage to look at the consequences dead on and don't try to hide behind excuses. Have you ever had someone apologize, and in the same sentence explain how it wasn't their fault and had nothing to do with them? That doesn't really feel like an apology at all, does it? On the other hand, have you ever had someone admit their mistake, own the outcome, and apologize sincerely? Feels much better, doesn't it?

When we get it right, when we admit our mistakes and own the consequences that come along with them, it allows everyone to move on rather than to get stuck. For example, when a boss makes an inappropriate racist or sexist comment, and then makes up a story about how it somehow wasn't their fault, no one can move on. We **have to** dig into what happened and make sure that a) they know that they were wrong, and b) it never happens again. If they don't admit their mistake, we have zero confidence in their ability to act differently next time. And bosses **require** the confidence of their workers in order to properly do their jobs.

When it goes right, we can move on because everyone is on the same page - we can at least have confidence that we share the same version of reality. If we don't do this, no one can move on because we can't trust that the mistake won't happen again. If we don't believe that our boss will keep a safe work environment for us or our coworkers, we cannot trust them enough to give the cooperation necessary for us to do our jobs. If we have a doctor who misdiagnosed us and led us down an incorrect treatment, and then didn't acknowledge the mistake, we can't trust them to do it right next time.

How it goes wrong

We've already done a lot of exploration of this – we get off track when our egos tell us to protect our sense of self by denying our mistakes. This can happen in a variety of different ways.

One phenomenon to particularly watch out for is convincing yourself that you are an exception.

For example: "I can't admit my mistake, I'm a leader/manager, and everyone will lose confidence in me." Or "You don't get it – In my field, you just *can't* make mistakes." Or "I don't think what I did was a mistake, but my wife clearly does!"

There are a million and one reasons why we weren't wrong. Why our shit doesn't stink as much as the next person's. Why we deserve a free pass on this one. Rather than argue against you, I want to remind you that there are no universal "shoulds" or imperatives here. There are just your choices and how you relate to them. I am not qualified to judge anyone on what happened or whether something was a mistake or not – it depends entirely on definitions.

The question is to you – what kind of person do you want to be? Do you want to take opportunities to grow and be a little less wrong than you once were? Or do you want to leave some of those opportunities behind? Again, not judging here – at the end of the day, you're the one who has to live with your choices. And as I've found, constantly living the path of growth can be incredibly exhausting.

If being human and making a mistake will lose you a relationship, a job, or an opportunity, I would propose that you ask yourself: If this relationship/job/opportunity requires me to be perfect and not make any mistakes at all, is that a condition that I'm willing to live with?

Understand that if you answer yes to that question, you are willingly signing yourself up for the consequences of your inevitable failure to be perfect all the time. And if the answer is no, I would invite you to renegotiate the terms. You might be surprised at what happens next – there are probably other humans in the situation who would also appreciate the chance to be human and not ostracized or punished for *their* mistakes.

Usually our relationship to mistakes "goes wrong" when we let our emotions or others' emotions sit in the driver's seat. We let our fear or upset about mistakes steer us down the wrong course. Emotions are absolutely essential in providing guidance, but I think you'll agree that they ought not to drive our decisions on their own, especially the important ones.

Pushing too hard

I mentioned in a previous story that I wrestled throughout high school. Wrestling was a fairly central part of my identity at the time. I identified very much with the struggle of it: with the exertion, the sweat, and the quest to prove myself. I was in the middle of the bell curve in terms of weight, which meant that my weight class typically had the most competitors in it. This meant that, in order to win a tournament, I would have to be the best out of between 16-32 wrestlers (sometimes even more), and wrestle 4-6 matches in a single day.

To give some perspective, a typical wrestling match involves nearly constant, maximum level exertion in all muscles in your body, for several minutes at a time without rest. Throw some adrenaline on top, along with the fear of being on display, and a sense that, if I lose in the ring, it means that I'm a failure as a person. Well, that's a recipe for disaster!

As a teenager, I had no idea that I didn't have to get so tied up emotionally in what I was doing. Every time I stepped in the ring, I had to prove myself by being the strongest, fastest, and best wrestler in my bracket. When it worked, and I won the tournament (which was rare - the competition was **fierce!**), my only reward was a temporary reprieve from the pressure. Which I couldn't really enjoy because I'd nearly wrestled myself into a coma. I wrestled like my life depended on it! Or at least, like my sense of self did.

One bad habit that I had picked up was to push hard into my opponents. I wasn't aware that I was doing it - I was so high-strung that I didn't notice much of anything. It was all a big, terrifyingly intense blur. My coach pointed out that I shouldn't lean in as hard, as it made me vulnerable to being thrown. Picture two people leaning hard into one another, and then one person switching in a microsecond from pushing to pulling - the one still pushing goes flying across the mat, usually to land on their back or even sail out of the ring (which happened more than a few times!) I would often lose matches this way.

Every time my coach pointed out to me that I was begging to be thrown with how I was standing and leaning, I would reflexively deny it. How could I acknowledge the criticism without also accepting that **I had caused my own loss?** My defensive teenaged brain, pushing back against all the pressure I felt to **get it right**, to **be enough**, couldn't accept the fact that I had made (and was continuing to make) a mistake. I kept denying it, and I kept getting thrown.

This pattern continued until one day, when I was wrestling in a great big tournament against the best wrestlers in the province. I was doing very well - I'd made it through a few rounds without losing yet. My coaches spotted the "guy to look out for" in my weight class - he'd recently wrestled in the even-bigger Canadian Finals, and ended up second place. In the whole country. I followed him closely, watching all of his matches to try to spot any weaknesses or patterns that I might exploit. He didn't give me much to work with. He was quick as lightning, and never seemed to tire or make mistakes. I knew I had my work cut out for me.

Eventually, we met in the ring and had an extremely intense match. I'm proud to say that I didn't lose right away!

We struggled back and forth in our epic encounter. At one point, I even had him on his back, until he wiggled us out of the ring, and we had to start again. Invigorated by my success, I started again very aggressively. I was in the lead, and just needed to score a few more points to end the match. I was out of my mind with adrenaline and the need to prove myself. I grabbed his arms, leaned in, and next thing I knew, I was flying through the air. My entire body was airborne, and my arms were trapped in his. I had no way of catching myself or softening the blow as I sailed above the head of my opponent and crashed with my weight combined with his weight, directly onto my head.

The world went black. I panicked and yelled out. I was terrified that I had broken my neck or something. My heartrate was probably through the roof. A few seconds later, my vision returned. Medics came to check that I was alright. They told me not to move. They checked my vision and reflexes. They checked my neck. Eventually, they asked if I was ok to continue the match. I said yes, but the truth was that I was already beaten. I got up and started wrestling again, but now I was behind in points, and in the end, I lost by a small margin. Small enough that if I had admitted my mistake long ago and stopped repeating it, I would have won.

I'd always felt able to brush my mistake under the carpet. To pretend I wasn't doing it. But that blackout terrified me. I was no longer able to pretend that I wasn't leaning in too hard. My brother (also a wrestler, and a very successful one) was there that day. I tried one last time to say that I didn't know how it had happened. He told me very frankly that I was pushing in way too hard. I respected his opinion, and I finally admitted the mistake.

Finally, I was able to start undoing the habit, and change how I wrestled. Admitting that mistake was the first step on the long path of learning to be a better wrestler. I learned how to turn the push to my advantage, by letting my opponent start to throw me and then counter it. None of this was possible until I accepted the flaw in my style.

I was foolish (aka, human) to deny that I had made a mistake. I didn't want to accept responsibility because I already felt crippling judgement for all my mistakes and failures - whether it was for not getting the top marks in all my classes, or not being the most popular kid, or even the failure of my silly high-school romances. Looking back, I realize that I had unthinkingly chosen values that were **very** dangerous and unnecessary.

Feeling the need to prove ourselves is a sure sign that we don't believe we're enough to begin with. If only I could ace this test, then I'll be alright. If only I could win this gold medal, I'll be enough. The problem with this is that it never ends. Never. No amount of accolades has the power to change our outlook. The only way to end the cycle is to stop participating. No amount of gold medals, friends, money, or anything else in this world will ever make us feel like we're enough. That's because feeling like enough comes from within, not from any of the external crap in this world.

How to come back

This is a skill set we're all going to need in our lives, at one point or another. For this one, I'm going to use a parenting example. As a parent, one is very often in the position of reacting to the mistakes of their children. How we react is very important, as it sets the stage for how our children will frame their mistakes in their own lives.

My wife is an excellent parent and most of what I know about how to deal with correcting children's mistakes has come from her. The strategy she uses is incredibly effective and, once you learn it, quite easy. Anytime our son Lewis (who is six years old as of the writing of this book) makes a mistake, she reacts by calmly but assertively pointing out that she'd like him to do something different than what he just did. Rather than making a big fuss about it, or using guilt or shame, she just corrects it, and nine times out of ten, the whole thing is resolved immediately. No fights, no arguments, no yelling, no hard feelings.

For example, Lewis will get too excited while playing and hit us a little too hard. She will say something like "Hey, you hit a little too hard there and it hurt. Can you try hitting a little softer next time?" Or "That didn't feel very good, can you be a bit more careful?" Or "I'm actually not enjoying the hitting, can we do a tickle fight instead?"

Behind her parenting is the assumption that Lewis isn't *trying* to hurt us or do the wrong thing. Even if he is, she makes a generous assumption of his motives that allows him to correct without all the negative emotion getting in the way. There is nothing inherently wrong or shameful about calibrating our behaviour, even if others would have us believe so.

Notice how the correction isn't "Hey, what the heck man? Why did you do that? What's wrong with you? What were you thinking?" Or "That was rude! You should have known better!" Or "That's it, I'm not playing with you anymore!"

Reacting in this second way puts children (and people in general) into a defensive mode and the issue quickly departs from the mistake itself and turns into a much deeper and more frightening topic – that the person is somehow inherently wrong for having done it. This is such an emotionally heavy prospect that children (and, again, people) have no choice but to push it away.

The first strategy can be hard to adapt if we're already accustomed to the second. Particularly if it's how *we* were parented. But if you think about it, the first strategy just makes sense, doesn't it? Correcting an unintentional mistake *should* be easy, matter-of-fact, and simple. It should be a simple observation and adjustment rather than a huge load of unnecessary and burdensome emotions.

Breaking out of the habit of confusing one's deeds with one's value as a person can be really tough, but in my experience, completely worth it.

Treating our own mistakes as my wife treats our child's mistakes, with compassion and useful corrective information, makes it much easier to move past them. I don't always get it right, but I try to follow her example, and whenever I do, I am always grateful to have chosen that approach. And I'm sure Lewis is as well.

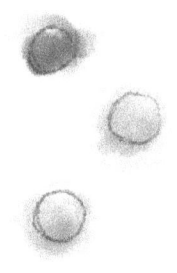

Part Three:
Celebrate!

The Power of Celebration

James is barrelling down the runway toward me, about to try a flip for the first time. My job is to stand next to the trampoline and make sure he makes it all the way around. Spotting acrobatic tricks is very difficult and requires one's full attention.

Unfortunately, I don't have that to give because I know that a fight is about to break out in the line-up. Again. James is approaching at a full sprint and I can't decide whether to stop him to address what's happening behind him or to keep my attention on him and help him through the jump.

We're at the Centre of Gravity circus school, and this is a regular occurrence for the vaulting part of our class. The unfortunate reality is that vaulting, by nature, is a one-person-at-a-time affair. Which is always a tricky prospect when you have 15 energetic, bouncing-off-the-walls children who want it to be their turn at all times.

*It was my least favourite activity to run because I hate to divide my attention away from the active child to address behavioural issues in the lineup. I say that it **was** my least favourite activity – it changed shortly after the session I was just speaking about.*

*Back to the gym – I decided to step in front of James and signal for him to stop. I then stalked angrily to the line-up and berated them for the hundredth time. As you may have guessed, the hundredth time was **not** the charm. The problem persisted until I had a breakthrough. My breakthrough came when, steeped in frustration after the class, I got to thinking about what makes circus fun. I realized that it's the action, the excitement, and the celebration.*

*But hang on – vaulting is totally action-packed! You get to run full speed, jump on a trampoline, and flip through the air to land on a big crash mat. How can you even **get** more exciting than that?*

*With more reflection, I realized that it wasn't the vaulting that made the kids act out. It was all the time **not** vaulting. They felt bored because they saw the vaulting as the activity, and all the time in between their turns as boring. I hadn't given* *them anything to fill the space between their turns. I reflected on all that I knew about what makes things fun, and decided to try something new. I decided to introduce a challenge.*

While the kids were waiting for their turns, I invited them to participate in a cheering competition. The competition was simple – whoever could cheer the loudest for the vaulting student would win.

What I saw was remarkable. It was as if someone had taken my old class away and given me a new one overnight. By the end of the next class, when James came barrelling down the runway, he had the energy of the entire group behind him, and boy, did he fly!

It took the students a while to warm up to the idea – at first they thought it was dumb. "Why should we cheer for him? Who cares?" They went through the motions half-heartedly at first. You can imagine kids pretending to be enthusiastic: "Oh yeah. Go James. Yeah. Great." It was forced, but at least they were doing it. And since they had their heads turned toward James, for the first time, they actually saw what James was working on. Then it was "Woah, hey, did you see that? That was actually pretty cool! Nice one James! Hey, how did you do that anyway? I want to do a flip too!"

Pretty soon, they were roaring with enthusiasm, and even their flops were celebrated, as they took mocking bows after a disgraceful faceplant to the thunderous cheers of their classmates. They were trying more ambitious tricks and not letting the fear of failure stop them – after all, a great flop sometimes leads to greater applause than a successful jump.

Eventually, they didn't even need me to egg them on, because they realized that it was so much more fun to be enthusiastic and cheer than to mope around being bored.

There were two main takeaways:
- *The group who was waiting was now having a great time. There were no fights or conflicts because everybody was busy cheering.*
- *The skill level of the students went through the roof (no pun intended...). Fueled by over-the-top encouragement and celebration from their friends, the vaulters stepped up*

their game and began learning more complex and more difficult tricks. We would have weekly vaulting high-jump competitions and for the first time I saw the students getting stronger and jumping higher. This opened new doors for more impressive jumps, which got more cheers and the whole thing snowballed.

This is the power of celebration. It transforms us from being bored, disengaged, and small to being open, expansive, and impressive. There is limitless energy in celebration, to be used however you choose. As long as you keep it positive, it will continue to flow, to branch out and make connections, to grow and bring us all together.

"Joy is in the ears that hear it"

This is one of my favourite quotes of all time, from one of my favourite authors, Stephen Donaldson. The statement is made by one of the Giants in Donaldson's Thomas Covenant series. The Giants always fascinated me. Their ability to find joy in everything, including misfortune, is what made them so compelling and different. It feels like an invitation to exist differently in the world than our normal western framework allows for. Our typical response to the world, especially adversity, is to battle, to control, to bend it to our will (or break ourselves in trying).

Our instinct toward this is often so deep that we don't even realize we have it. We simply act according to our story of *having to make things right all the time*, and we don't even realize the costs because we're not acquainted with another framework. The Giants in Donaldson's story provide us with that framework. Their indomitable will springs directly from their connection to the joy in everything. Their lives are lived in the joy of service to the beauty they see in absolutely everything, even darkness. And their power lies in their service to the world around them. Each feat spurs them on to another feat, for sheer joy of the possibility of it.

I believe that this spirit identified by Donaldson is present in all of us as humans. I think that we all have the same capacity for joy, incredible accomplishments, and service to our world, and we are limited only by the framework we've chosen to adopt. Please note that when I speak of the limitations of our capacities, I'm not speaking of external limitations. I recognize that, as an able-bodied white male in

North America, I have the privilege of pursuing and achieving just about anything. I also recognize that many people in the world will never have the opportunities I have for the simple fact of where & to whom they were born.

The world of circus is a direct embodiment of a powerful framework. It's our raw potential, put into action with incredible feats that defy our perceived limits, in joy and in celebration. Circus arts are a structured and deep pursuit of human capabilities that are specifically designed to bring us joy. They are a beautiful representation of making our dreams come true. And, just as with dreams, circus has this miraculous power to *surprise us*. To introduce a new and radically different experience that we couldn't even have imagined.

Circus forces us to stretch our old frameworks to accommodate its incredible feats. Something you would have sworn to be impossible, performed right in front of you, is proof that your expectations, your framework, is incorrect. And it does it with elegance and joy – you can adjust your idea without having to feel like an idiot.

How does it have this power? Because it's a celebration, dammit! The whole point of it is to enjoy ourselves! To escape the "life is work" mentality, and take in something new, unexpected, and delightful. It tells us that we're wrong about how we're living, in the nicest possible way. That is, that life really is a celebration, and if celebrating gives us more power in the world by amplifying the impact of our actions, what the hell else are we doing with our time?!

Now before you come back to me with a "Hey Andrew, but what about all the suffering out there? How can I find joy when my life (and/or others') are a trainwreck?!", I want to elaborate a little bit. First, I want to recognize that, as far as external circumstances are concerned, I've had it pretty damn good in my life. I'm extremely privileged in more ways that I can count. I've never had to deal with the external hardships that many others have to face. I wouldn't dare condescend to say that I know anything about going through the struggles others have gone (and are still going) through. But I believe that what I have to say transcends that.

See, I believe that our experiences on the inside really don't have to match what's happening on the outside. In fact, I think that all external hardships only count as hardships because they cause us to feel uncomfortable on the inside. There are countless examples of this: trekking up a mountain may be extreme hardship for one person and an extremely rewarding adventure for another. Eating fifty-six hotdogs in one sitting can be a triumph for one person and a horrible ordeal for another.

There's no inherent link between our happiness and specific circumstances - a bad breakup is only painful insofar as it gives us painful emotions. We've probably had plenty of times being happy *without* our partner, and plenty of times being unhappy even *with* our partner. Our circumstances and are emotions are less entwined than we seem to think. Breakups are only hardships if they make us deal with a painful emotional landscape on the inside. That is, it's not the loss of a partner that sucks - it's the emotions that we are forced to feel as a result. Losing your job is only a hardship if it makes you feel emotions about money or your coworkers or something else. I can think of at least 3 jobs that I am much happier to be without.

For one of the most profound and eloquent accounts of the discrepancy between internal and external experience, read Viktor Frankl's "Man's Search for Meaning". Frankl is a holocaust survivor who witnessed and experienced some of the absolute worst external circumstances, living in a concentration camp. Physical and psychological abuse were just the beginning – there was also disease, starvation, people freezing to death, things we would rather not imagine. And yet, in the midst of such suffering and external hardship, Frankl witnessed both guards and prisoners deriving a sense of meaning from treating each other with dignity, kindness, and generosity. Sharing moldy hunks of bread even when on the verge of total starvation, sharing ratty scraps of blankets with sick comrades. Frankl writes about how all of this is possible even in those terrible times.

Another example comes to mind of a profound disparity between internal and external circumstances I read recently. It was a career profile on a man in Haiti whose job it is to clean out public latrines. By hand. With no safety equipment. And no, I'm not making this up. He had to literally wade into pits, filled usually up to the top of his head with public sewage, and empty them somehow. Every day.

To be honest, it doesn't actually surprise me much that this job exists – there are a lot of really poor people in very densely populated places in the world, and *someone* has to get the job done. And if they're so poor that they don't have the proper equipment, well, it just means someone has to get real dirty.

No, what was really noteworthy about this story was that the man was **proud to have his job**. He got a lot of pride from working hard in service of his community, doing a job that most would be unable to do, and in the meantime, he could feed his damn family! He decided that, even though the job is so obviously unpleasant, that's not nearly as important as his ability to feed his family, and by paying the costs to do this, he won a sense of pride. Yes, it was nasty, and yes, he got sick often, but what's the alternative? To starve to death? To do it but hate yourself for doing it? What the hell kind of alternatives are those?

I'll bet that his pride in his ability to do his job was directly proportional to the suffering he carried to be able to do it. The more he had to work for it, the more those rewards meant. Now, while this might not look like it, this man is engaged in a form of celebration. **He's exercising his ability to act in service of the things he feels are important.** I would venture to say that this is where meaning is generated for *all of us*.

So here he is, with some pretty nasty external circumstances, but a pretty rich inner experience (I'm inferring, based on his words). Even though he's literally covered in shit almost all the time, he's happy and fulfilled. And yet, even though most of us have much better external circumstances than our Haitian friend, we probably can't claim so much internal satisfaction and joy.

Take me on the other hand. I was born in a loving, middle-class family with a rich culture and every opportunity to succeed. I never had to worry about not having enough food, or being safe. I got so many chances to do things that others will never have. And, despite all of that, a significant portion of my life was characterised by intense internal suffering.

In fact, for a number of years, my entire external world was almost completely eclipsed by my internal experience of suffering. I mentioned in the introduction about learning that I had an anxiety disorder. I'd like to explain a little more about that now.

Anxious about "nothing"

I was very excited to finally be attending university, escaping my high school world. I had assumed that this would be the end of petty judgements, small-minded social groups, and the constant pressure to "get it right". I didn't realize that, even though I was escaping that particular group of people, the university campus would be filled with others who had come from their own high schools, and would be bringing their own high school culture with them. Or that the pettiness of high school is actually pretty typical of how much of the world works.

I quickly realized that university life had largely the same set of social challenges as high school – how do I fit in? How do I find a group who will be supportive of me and my interests rather than cruel and judgemental? Am I still going to be ostracized for not being part of the jocks & "popular kids"?

Nope, people, by and large, were really not much more mature in university than they were in high school, only I didn't have a place to escape anymore. Rather than being able to go home at the end of the day, I was stuck in a residence with people I didn't get along with. In a double room about the size of a closet.

I recall memories such as wanting to sleep at three in the morning but having no option to do so, with 50 people crammed into my room that's designed for 2, crowded around a small fish tank in the centre of the room, hollering at the top of their lungs, cheering for the fish fighting to the death in the bowl. And yes, there were 50 – I counted because I had nothing else to do at the time.

Or another time when I wanted nothing more than to sleep, and instead had a front row seat to what was probably the most Neanderthal competition I've ever seen – the guys from my section taking turns whacking a leftover plastic devil's trident from Halloween on each other, comparing the size of the ensuing welts. In my room. In the middle of the night.

Clearly, this was no paradise I had escaped to. I didn't have very many friends during my time there – looking back, I think I had assumed that the whole university population shared the strange values I witnessed in those late-night residence "parties", which I wanted nothing to do with. So I mostly kept to myself. So much so that it started to get dangerous.

I started telling myself the story that I was alone, and by second year (when I finally had a room to myself), I stopped leaving my house unless I had to. And the less I left, the less I *wanted to leave. The less I felt like I **could** leave. I was trapped in a horrible paradox – **needing** to connect with other human beings, yet too terrified to try.*

*I internalized it all, and started believing myself **unworthy** of human company. It didn't seem dramatic or an overreaction at the time – I really **was** quite different from most of those around me, and most of my significant experiences were of people mocking or rejecting me for not being like them. And as much as I wanted to not care about it, I didn't realize how deeply humans need to belong to a group.*

I spiralled down and down into a pretty deep pit of self-hatred and anxiety. Leaving my house was so dangerous because it was another chance for the world to confirm to me that I didn't belong. I couldn't take that chance because it was too painful to have my sense of self constantly dashed on the rocks of others' judgements.

My anxiety grew and grew to the extent that I could now point to it and say "See? There's the proof that there's something wrong with me! Look, I can't even walk into a classroom because I can't stand to have people look at me! This is proof that I don't belong here." My dysfunction was palpable and unavoidable – even though I tried as if my life depended on it (and it really did), I just couldn't shake the thoughts or feelings. Ignoring it didn't work – if I tried to go out to the bar as my housemates urged me to, I would just end up in a big mess and feel like I had utterly betrayed myself. As if I had knowingly stuck my hand in the fire. I hated myself for my betrayal, and then doubly so for the feelings of anxiety that kept me from enjoying myself around others.

I hated myself so badly that I developed addictions. One was to marijuana, which sometimes provided me the opportunity to immerse myself in tasks that made me forget my anxiety, and sometimes made it worse. The other was a process of self-improvement through self-destruction. I would train and work out in ways that were definitely not healthy.

I would take out my rage on myself by training far past my limits – I would create real pain in my body to match the emotional pain I couldn't get rid of. And it was all fueled by my hatred for my own weakness. As if I could burn it out of me and use the heat to galvanize myself into a better version of myself that was immune to the pain of isolation.

One day, I had an important class to go to, so I got on the bus to get to school. It was already precarious for me to leave the house, but when I set foot on the bus, things got real intense.

*I remember the sudden sense of complete panic as all the eyes on the bus were on me. Walking down the aisle of the bus, I was convinced that something was wrong. Deeply wrong. In my head, I went through a horrible checklist to explain why everyone was looking at me. "Is my fly down? Did I remember to wear clean clothes today? Are my shoelaces untied? Why is everyone looking at me? What's going on? Can they tell that I'm panicking here? Oh my god, they can tell, can't they? Just act normal. How the hell do I do that?! What do I do? How do I stop panicking? What the hell is wrong with me? I can't even get on a bus without freaking out! Jesus, look at everyone else, they're totally normal, why can't I just feel like that even once?! Oh shit, now I'm breathing too fast. Why can't I catch my breath? Oh god, now everyone is **really** starting at me, I need to get out of here!"*

*I ended up pulling the cord and getting out at the very next stop. I was too embarrassed to go to class after that, so I turned around and walked right back home. And the next time, I was that much less likely to even **try** taking the bus. Or being around people. My research (for the very class I was too anxious to go to – Abnormal Psychology) told me that I was experiencing anxiety attacks. And if you've never had one, let me tell you – they're goddamn awful. Bad enough that you can easily justify just about any strategy to avoid the possibility of having another one. Even if it means total isolation.*

Again, my external circumstances were actually fine. I wasn't starving, I was in no physical danger, I wasn't at risk of being killed because of the colour of my skin or my political views. I wasn't homeless, and my family was alive and well. I didn't have money to spare, but I also never had to worry about paying my rent or buying food. I wasn't struggling with cancer or a physical disability. I wasn't being abused, and I never had to live in fear of the police, gangs, crime, or really anything at all. My life on the outside was as good as one could reasonably expect. But it didn't feel that way **at all**. It seemed unbearable – the world represented a big, scary, overwhelming force that rarely brought me anything but pain and suffering.

All of this is to say that, while I am lucky enough to have had one of the highest rolls of the dice in terms of external life, that doesn't mean that I've had the best internal life. I've spent a lot of time in some *very* dark places. And I'll bet a lot of you have too. The reason that I do the work that I do, and the reason I am writing this book is to give another option of a perspective for those who have experienced or are still experiencing something similar.

So, if we're stuck in a dark awful pit of self-loathing or anxiety, or whatever it is, how can we even *imagine* something preposterous like celebrating? What the hell is there to celebrate if we feel like absolute garbage all the damn time? Well, the good news is that, **if our internal world is divorced from our external world, we don't ever have to wait for things to change**. We don't need that new car/attractive partner/flashy new outfit because those things are just incidental anyway! Not only are they "easy-come-easy-go", but they also don't matter nearly as much as we think they do. A single pebble may mean more to us than a sports car, as long as we can hold the possibility that it can. I acknowledge that cultivating that kind of mindframe is far from easy, but hey - as far as I'm concerned, it's the only game in town!

I'd like to revisit Anthony from chapter 1. Remember - he was born without normally functioning arms. And he still learned to juggle. Rather than spending his time moping and complaining about the limitations of his body, he was fully engaged in doing the things that his body **is** capable of doing. That, my friends, is celebration. It's taking what you've got and saying it's enough. No, it's more than enough. It's a bounty that is worth paying tribute to. And that tribute looks different for each of us, as it should. For Anthony, in that moment, it was juggling. For me, it's just about anything that's in front of me.

To tell the truth, I find just about everything interesting and worth doing. I wish I could live a thousand lifetimes just to explore and pay tribute to all of the incredible things around me. There are so many books I would read, so many activities I would do, so many skills I would learn. Why? Because I can! And so can most of you. So, I ask – what gets in the way of celebrating for you?

I heard of a saying once: "Only boring people are bored." I like it. The point is essentially that the things themselves aren't boring

– it's your approach to them. Boringness is to be found in *you*, not in the things around you. If you set yourself up with the expectation that the world around you ought to bend over backwards to make itself interesting and entertain you in every moment, you'll always come back to boredom. Because there will inevitably be that moment when the Youtube video you're watching just doesn't have enough flashing lights, or your data runs out, or the person in front of you isn't telling you the absolute most interesting thing you've ever heard in your life in their current sentence.

I'm serious – it's a bad place to be! Have you ever had the pleasure of interacting with someone who is perpetually bored? It seems so unpleasant, doesn't it! It's like you have to crank up the dial on everything that comes out of your mouth just so that they will pay attention and not check their phone in the middle of what you're saying. Do you think their strategy is serving them?

This fallacy of believing that it's up to the world to entertain us and that we have no obligation to create, only to consume, leaves us unfulfilled and constantly in judgement. We're putting ourselves in this role where we are literally *always* looking for flaws and other things that we don't like about what's in front of us. It's as if, in the background of absolutely every moment, we're sitting on the fence, asking ourselves: "Is it still worth my attention now? How about now? Now? Now? Now?" We're not truly giving ourselves in *any* moment, and this leaves us purposeless and without joy.

With the unlimited amounts of entertainment and information that are available at a moment's notice in our pockets or in our hands, we've forgotten our role in seeing the value of what's in front of us.

A great friend of mine once described this judgemental frame of mind with an analogy of continually cranking up the volume on life, while we've got our fingers plugging our ears and bragging about how loud it can be and still not affect us. Or like saying "Hey, check out how much beauty I can be blind to! Watch how unimpressed I can be! Aren't I great?!" Which is a really bizarre thing to do, don't you think? Especially if you do it every day about everything you experience, and then wonder why nothing means anything to you. It's because you're blocking it out! You've got your fingers in your ears and you wonder why nothing makes it through to you. Just take your fingers out of your ears, man! Stop dismissing things after a quarter of a second of boredom. I promise that the world is full of beautiful and interesting things, you just have to stop judging and rejecting it all!

"Interesting people are interested."

There's another way to be, another answer to the question of how to relate to what's around us. That is, to see the miracle and boundless horizons of everything around us. Each thing, no matter how trivial, actually has a great depth to it if you're willing to explore. I am fortunate enough to have a few great models of this idea in my life. Everything from the smallest nuts and bolts (literally – have you ever seen how those things are made? Absolutely fascinating!) to the biggest mountains has more depth to it than you could ever learn in a lifetime of study.

The world in a bucket

Time for a thought exercise: Let's take a totally trivial example. Let's pick a bucket. You might look at a bucket and say "So what? It's a bucket." Did you know that buckets are incredibly deep (ha!)? And yes, I'm serious. I had the privilege of watching an hour-long documentary of a master cooper at work. Cooper is the job title of someone who makes buckets, barrels, and other containers of the sort. You probably think buckets are simple – they're round and they hold stuff like water. Well, how do you think we did that in the age before plastic?

That's what a cooper would do – he (during the early days of manufacturing, almost every single tradesperson was a "he" {another fascinating sub-point – why would this be? Are men inherently any more able to make buckets or any other things than women? What were the political, social, and economic conditions that gave rise to this?}) would have to carve (using only hand tools - no machinery, that would come later) each piece of the bucket to be exactly identical, with exactly the correct angle to each of its sides. Buckets are angled out from the bottom to the top – this is part of what gives it the structural integrity to hold its shape under pressure.

The cooper would have to calculate each of these compound angles (without a calculator – that also, is to come later), and then measure and cut each stave (that's what the planks of a bucket or barrel are called) to be exactly right, without a protractor. This process takes **hours***, even for a master cooper. After the staves are cut just right, the bottom needs to be cut. Did you know that it needs to be a slight oval, with the wide part being across the grain of the wood? It's because the woodgrain compresses width-wise over time, and if you don't make it a slight oval, even your perfectly made, seaworthy bucket will leak within a year or two. And most people don't like leaky buckets.*

With sides and bottom cut, it's time to make the metal rings that wrap around the staves to hold them in place. Each one has to be custom-measured and cut – no cheating and pre-fabricating here! The process goes on and on, to a much greater depth than I've just described. And I haven't even gotten into the kinds of wood you need to use here, that will swell when wet to prevent leaks, or how it is prepared before the cooper even gets it (obviously there can't be any cracks, but would you know how to transform a tree into lumber of the right dimensions and moisture content without it cracking?), or what tools the cooper uses, and how each of them are made.

We haven't cracked into barrels yet – how one would calculate the size, roundedness, number of pieces, or angle of cuts to make a barrel. Imagine – someone tells you to make them a barrel to hold 200 gallons of wine. Where would you even start with your calculations? Did your math class ever cover how to calculate the volume of a bloated cylinder? I thought not. And I'll bet the cooper never even went to a single damn math class in his life! So how on earth did he learn how to make the pieces to make a barrel that'll hold precisely 200 gallons? Keep in mind that, in the age of the cooper, almost all goods were transported by barrel. That meant that it wasn't just one obscure dude who made all the barrels. It was an army of them! Each one closely guarding their own secret formulas for calculating and making the barrels, their own "trade secrets".

You can see how even the humble bucket can be the pursuit of a lifetime of inquiry, and you'll never get to the bottom of it. Even the subject of the bucket leaks at its edges into every other discipline and inquiry. We saw math, woodworking, tool fabrication, economics, history, socio-political analysis already in my brief description.

We could easily expand into the domains of human strength and biomechanics of the actions of actually making the parts, anatomy, language, business, forestry, climate history, cellular structure, and on and on and on. How about metal buckets? Plastic buckets? Glass buckets? Ok, there probably aren't glass buckets, but I'll bet you could write a whole essay on why glass buckets would be a bad idea by analysing the molecular structure of glass, incorporating economics, fabrication techniques, etc. etc. etc.

In case you're having trouble seeing how the subject of buckets being endlessly deep ties into celebration, let me make the link for you. I will bet that before reading the passage above, most of you had completely dismissed "buckets" as being totally uninteresting, and never stopped to think any further. You probably never considered a single one of the things we just went through together. I'll bet that you thought it was a dead end, so you stopped looking. In fact, I'll bet that you do that about a **lot** of things. And when I say a lot of things, I mean almost everything. You think it's a dead end and so you dismiss it. You figure that there are better things to do with your time.

A bucket (or anything else) is only a dead end *because* we stop looking. We think it's up the world to be an endless parade of the most interesting things conceivable, and we forget our role in the whole thing. When we do this, we cease to celebrate. We sit back with our arms crossed, imperiously shouting "Next! Next! Next!", as if any of it has the power to penetrate our self-imposed walls. We don't realize that each discipline, each pursuit, each subject, is infinitely complex and nuanced, and can captivate the interested mind for as long as it might want. You just have to exit your well-constructed castle of judgement and explore the world as it is. And when you do, you realize that there really *is* nothing special about you that makes you any better than a cooper, or anyone else who does one of the myriad things you've dismissed.

If you think about it, you'll realize that something isn't either interesting or uninteresting in itself - it is YOU that makes it so.

Being able to see the beauty, the depth, the nuance, in things, is a gift. It literally transforms the world in front of our very eyes. In the space of a moment, a hallway of closed doors can fly open and you can feel the boundless depth of value in absolutely everything around you. The best part of the gift is that it is available to each of us in every moment, if we choose to be open to reaching out and experiencing it. You don't have to *earn it*. All you have to do is just stop shutting it out.

As I say this, you may find your mind coming back to the following rebuttal: "Ok, sure - But what about all the people who don't have the luxury of spending their time contemplating buckets? What about people with deep and serious challenges that a change in mindset can't get rid of?" It's a fair point. Maybe you find yourself in that category. I will continue to acknowledge my privileged position in having the time and resources to be able to write a book about the philosophy of juggling.

I will also respond by pointing out that it's human nature to feel like we need to change what's in front of us rather than changing *how we see* what's in front of us. The truth is that they are completely separate pursuits, and we're far more inclined to do the former than the latter. That is, we're far more inclined to attribute our emotions in any given moment, to what's going on outside of us rather than what's going on inside of us. And therefore, we're far more likely to direct our efforts to changing the world around us rather than changing ourselves.

Let me be clear - I'm not bashing this strategy. Not at all. Sometimes, the biggest challenge for us really *is* on the outside – having to deal with a toxic work or home environment can have a huge impact on us. But it's dangerous when we use *only this strategy* and never look inside when it comes to making changes. Because I believe that it's incomplete without also looking inside.

Changing the world requires changing ourselves - remember that quote: "Be the change you wish to see in the world"? If we already had the skills to make the world different, we would have done so already, wouldn't we? The fact that the world remains how it is, is proof that we've still got work to do on the inside. And I believe that a vital part of that work is the shift in perspective I'm trying to describe.

When we wear the right set of eyes, we'll never have to waste our effort in continuing to change what's in front of us because it will all be beautiful. Even the suffering.

Did Anthony stop and question whether juggling was worth his time? No! He just did it for the simple fact that he could, and he rocked it! And I'll bet that he took his success and snowballed it into the next thing he did, and so on and so on. Each rewarding exploration empowers us to take on more adventures, to explore more divergent paths. Some people (myself included) have saved themselves on a deep level from very painful lives by finding the joy of celebration. Some of my students have transformed their lives in profound ways through celebrating the learning and exhibition of skills they never had before. Let's pause here for a quick example of one:

What it looks like

Beauty is in the eyes of the beholder

I still remember the precise moment that I met Garrett. I was juggling for some nervous new students at the Centre of Gravity Circus School, and before he even walked into the gym, I heard him:

"WOOOOOOOAAAAAHHHH!!! That is SOO COOL! How can you DO THAT?! WOAH! COOL! Do that again! Again!"

*He was totally in awe of what he was seeing, and I was caught off guard. I didn't think I was **that** good at juggling. I actually wondered if he was being sarcastic and making fun of me. One look at his face told me he was being sincere – his eyes were wide and filled with wonder. It was quite endearing actually – I felt like I had my own personal cheerleader in the class.*

Garrett, I learned, has autism. He is unaware of how he comes across to others, a characteristic that made his life difficult at times. As I got to know him more, his parents told me that he had a lot of trouble connecting with his peers because, like many with autism, he doesn't have the social skills that most of us take for granted. He would get mocked for being sincere and open-hearted the way he did on his first day. It breaks my heart to think of how common this experience is among kids – getting ostracized for caring about things.

As Garrett came to more and more of our programs and summer camps, he had a singular focus on learning the skills that a lot of the other students were much more casual about. It paid off for Garrett in a BIG way. He learned to juggle very quickly, became quite good at acrobatics, and even taught himself to ride a unicycle (I actually had no part in that at all!). He was quite delightful to be around, as he loved to share the joy of his exploration with those around him. He was so thrilled to be doing what he was doing that it was infectious.

As his coach at the circus school, I only ever got to see Garrett in his element, learning new skills and having a great time. What I didn't realize was how transformative this experience was for Garrett in his life outside of the school. I learned that his journey in circus transformed his identity from being the awkward kid who never really fit in, to a celebrity, admired wherever he went. His parents told me about what a huge step it was for Garrett's independence. He used to hate going to school because he felt so awkward around his peers.

Now, he was riding his unicycle around town, completely on his own! Mastering that skill even gave him the confidence to introduce himself to total strangers (something he had never previously done). The fact that he was riding a unicycle around town acted as an icebreaker and gave him an easy way to start conversations. Conversations that his circus skills gave him the confidence to have. In celebrating his capacity to learn these skills, Garrett himself became the object of celebration.

To me, Garrett always looked like a star. Right from the first moment he walked in our doors, he was uplifting to be around, and always gave a sincere effort to anything, even if it was difficult and his peers would give up. But the sad reality is that Garrett's life outside of circus school wasn't that way at all. Garrett was not set up to succeed in his life outside of our little circus bubble. Between an educational system that deplores individuality, peers who mock failure, and a harsh, success-driven culture, Garrett was shuffled offstage.

Garrett's "transformation" didn't look at all like a transformation to me. It just looked like an awesome kid being awesome. And it got me thinking – isn't this what we could *all* be like if we just found our own version of circus arts? Sure, Garrett and I come alive when we're on our unicycles or juggling or whatever else, but I recognize that unicycles and juggling aren't for everyone. I think that there are almost as many outlets for human spirit and celebration as there are people in this world. Maybe more!

As long as we don't get too fixated on what celebrating *should* look like, I believe we'll all be able to find our own version of celebration. Something that calls us to be alive, to throw ourselves into our work/play in a way that we don't care so much about "failing" or not meeting others' expectations. Some people write poems, some people make cheese, some people sing, dance, or create puzzles. Some people do them all at the same time! Well, maybe not. But hey - you could be the first!

It can be tempting to believe that to do this is selfish. That pursuing our interests, celebrating what makes us come alive, is somehow wrong. You might say "Andrew, I'd love to be eating cheese all day, but what the hell good is that going to do in our world?" Well, I believe that true celebration doesn't mean sitting at the back of the room, arms greedily clutching the cheese tray as you shove it all in your mouth.

What I have seen, time and again, across every field, is that, when people *truly* come alive in celebration, *they have no choice but to share it*. Rather than seeing it as an "indulgence", those invested in the practice of celebrating are *constantly* sharing their passion with others. They are the ones going out of their way to give their joy, and the joy of their craft, to the world around them. They're the ones who start community groups, the ones who teach beginners for free, the ones who start foundations and travel and bring their craft across the world. They're the ones writing books, making videos, burning with a desire to give, to share, to help others come alive the way they have.

The Cheese Ambassador

To keep with our example of cheese, I want to share a quick story. I had the privilege of meeting an interesting colleague this past year at the Canadian Association of Professional Speakers (CAPS) annual convention. His name is David Beaudoin, and he's the Canadian Cheese Ambassador. That means that his job is to serve the cheese industry by educating the public, leading cheese tastings, working with Canadian cheese farmers, creating community, sharing best practices, etc. He loves his work so much that his enthusiasm is contagious.

> *I went to one of David's cheese tastings, and it was apparent within moments that he was exactly the right person to be leading it. It was clear that he was hosting the event because he loves cheese so much that he delights in giving others the experience of discovering new flavours and textures.*
>
> *Frankly, I can't think of a better person to be leading people through the process of cheese tasting. It was truly a pleasure to get to experience his passion for delicious Canadian cheeses. I didn't, even for a second, think of David as self-centred or self-indulgent. Because that's not how he acted – he was generous and enthusiastic, and truly cared about our having a good time. He truly **was** a cheese ambassador.*

I think that David's example and particularly his job title gives us a great way of thinking about celebrating. In having and exploring our passions, we become "ambassadors". We care what people think about them because we experience so much joy from them that we can't help but want others to have the same experience of joy.

Celebrating our interests with humility and dedication fills us with so much joy that we can't even contain it all – we are overflowing with such abundance that we leave our scarcity mindset behind, and find enough left over that the whole world can have a slice. Furthermore, it becomes *our job* to share a slice with everyone in the world.

Taking on this task, the task of sharing our celebration, requires us to grow. It pushes us in the best possible way. It invites us to step out of our old shell of living to survive, and points the way to something better. We transcend our old selves, and do things we never would have dreamed of doing. Our horizons expand as our passions bring us to new places.

We learn more about ourselves, stepping into the inheritance we are all born with – the endless beauty of what's around us. We also learn more about others – we must, in order to understand how to translate our joy for what's in front of us to those we want to share with. Our focus shifts beyond ourselves as we learn to serve something greater than ourselves. We no longer care so much about serving our smaller personal perspective, and attune ourselves to something deeper, something wider.

Celebrating, by acting in service of the things we care about, the things that make us come alive (by allowing ourselves to *believe it's possible*, and by allowing ourselves to *drop the ball*), gives us a kind of superpower. The best way I can describe it is like drinking from a fountain that represents the wellspring of all energy.

Some people believe that no such fountain exists, or perhaps that it has dried up. Perhaps you find yourself in that camp. They watch the dry faucet and claim that there *is* no boundless stream gushing infinitely from it's spout, not realizing that they have unknowingly closed the spigot.

Remember the boredom mindset - the constant demanding of the world to give us more, more more? That's a sure sign that we've closed ourselves off. For some, there are only meager drops intermittently escaping the spout, but I believe that this, too, is caused by our closing the taps in ignorance and unawareness. It can be hard to believe that we would do this, and therefore easy to dismiss or contradict this explanation.

I don't think that anyone does this knowingly – that anyone would willfully cut themselves off from the boundless stream of spirit energy. There's a whole lot to us beneath the surface that we either don't think is important, or are too afraid to really look at. And even if we are willing and able to explore the depths of ourselves to find how we might be doing this, the parts of ourselves that are responsible for closing our wellsprings are really good at hiding. Don't forget – they have access to our story-making abilities and powers of justification too!

We can deny or justify these parts of ourselves all day long, and I have no business engaging in that with you. All I can do is invite you to truly look at whether you may be precluding yourself from this life of celebration, either consciously or unconsciously.

That's all this book is – an invitation to what I believe is a better way of life, that in my experience seems to be universally accessible to all human beings. It is up to you whether or not you accept my invitation and come play in what is sometimes a scary, unknown jungle, or to stay in the comfort of your home, and forever be at the mercy of what happens around you.

Feel free to think of some people that you admire who are engaged in celebration of some sort. Perhaps they show excellence in bringing people together, in some skilled trade or craft. Perhaps they are pursuing frontiers that have never been explored before and bringing their knowledge to the world.

One point of distinction that I want to make, about what

celebrating *doesn't* look like: using your object of celebration to feel more important than others. Our egos can very easily construct our reality to make it seem like we are somehow better for being so knowledgeable about our own personal "cheese".

Anytime you find yourself ranking yourself in relation to others, you're not really celebrating. Remember that true celebration requires keeping your object of celebration as being *higher than yourself*. True celebration is about service – staying a humble beginner sharing what little part we have come to know about our passion.

How it goes wrong

I believe that there are three significant ways that we stray from the path of celebration
- Living in disharmony with ourselves
- Letting our ego take over
- Evaluating & judging ourselves and others

Living in disharmony with ourselves

How exactly does one unknowingly close the spigot of energy in their lives? The truth is, there are a million and one ways, and I'm only just starting to understand and recognize the ways I do it in my own life. One of the most common things I've seen (in myself and in others) is denying that such a spigot exists, or that there are parts of ourselves that operate without our awareness, that preclude our access without our knowing.

The Underworld

Here's another thought experiment. To describe how we do this, I want to use an analogy that has been very helpful to me in my journey of discovery. Imagine your life represented by the Earth. The landscape represents your unique patterns, your propensities and gifts, your faults and limitations. We each have our deserts, our fertile plains, our wild jungles, our steep cliffs and our deep seas. You can work with them or against them, but they're there regardless of how you feel about them or how you relate to them. This is your starting point.

Everything you've built in your life can be represented by the buildings on your planet. Some are small and modest, others may be grand and impressive. Some stand tall while others are closer to ground. Some of the things you've done crumble and fall apart in time – some are washed away by the rising tide, whereas others are enduring. Some are functional and others are purely decorative. Maybe you tried tennis a few times but it didn't last. Maybe you've been knitting your whole life. The former would be a forgotten old building, and the latter would be a bustling metropolis.

The landscapes and buildings, everything you can see on the surface represents your "conscious" life. That is, every story, every event, every encounter, every building, and every facet of the landscape, lies on the surface of your life. That's all that we can really see or know in our conscious minds. It would be tempting to look at all this and conclude that that's all there is. After all, we've built so much, we've had so many stories, we can look easily at it all and see the edges, where everything begins and ends. It is easily defined and you can take out your measuring tape and see how it all stacks up and relates to each other thing.

However, I believe that there's a whole other world beyond what's on the surface. This world is rich and unfathomably deep. In fact, it runs so deep that you could spend your entire life digging, and never get to the core. And when we explore this way, we find that the things beneath the surface are strange and hard to wrap our heads around. They don't look like anything we've ever seen on the surface, and we're not quite sure what to do with them. They defy our understanding and puzzle us.

We're tempted to use our surface-level understanding to explain them, but they never quite fit into our meaning system. We have to ignore parts of what we see in order for them to be understandable. We experience such wacky and unbelievable things that we often throw them out wholesale, as if our ability to believe them or not is a valid measure of whether they exist. Believe it or not, our minds are chock full of crazy stuff that doesn't make sense, that we have a really hard time seeing or accepting. These are the underground denizens that we all, *like it or not, carry with us.*

To flip back to a concrete example, imagine that you are hesitant to try to juggle because something beneath the surface in your life tells you not to. Your conscious mind doesn't understand what part of you is saying this or why, but its job is to keep it all making sense. So you come up with a reason: "Oh, my wrist hurts today." Or "I can't do it, don't bother wasting your time on me." Or "I'm feeling tired." But those are never really the reasons, are they?

I want to take a moment to cite an experiment that illustrates how our conscious minds have the persistent habit of justifying our actions after we're acted, and then fully buy into our BS explanation of why we did that thing. I heard about this experiment some time ago, so forgive me if I'm missing a detail or two.

The jist of it is that experimenters artificially stimulated the motor cortex in the brain of the participant to induce them to move their leg. They would then ask the participant why they did it, and they would, in every single case without fail, come up with some reason why **they chose to do it** (and fully believe their own explanation!) Even though they knew exactly what the premise of the experiment was, they really truly believed that moving their leg was their own choice, and not the result of their brain getting zapped. They acted, and their rational mind was confused (presumably by the fact that it was a novel experience), and so it had to come up with an explanation about why they chose to do it. Their explanations would sound something like "Oh, my leg was falling asleep, I had to move it." Or "It was starting to feel awkward so I had to adjust." Or "I just felt like it". In fact, I heard that the head researcher, who designed the experiment, was so baffled that he insisted on being a participant himself. When his assistants hooked him up and jolted his brain to move his leg, he too insisted that it was his own choice! Isn't that wild?

Our surface minds, presided over by our egos, want to feel like they're in control. And I mean REALLY want to be in control. So much so that they invent the illusion of control even when it is obviously impossible. Just ask an addicted gambler why they continue to gamble. Even when they understand their own logical fallacies (like the one where past losses somehow *increase future chances of winning), they still buy into them because they require that illusion of control.*

Our desire for control strongly resists situations where we lose control, which explains why we're so reluctant to explore the parts of ourselves that we can neither explain nor control. The overwhelming feeling we get when we explore deeper than the surface of our lives is confusion. We're not sure if we're really seeing it or not. Maybe we're making it up. We must be – the things we find down there don't make any sense, are illogical and inconsistent. Every time we think we've properly classified them, they change, mutate, slip away, and we're left empty-handed and wondering.

Our conscious minds will never be able to properly classify them because they don't follow the rules of the things on the surface. In the times when we encounter our deeper parts, our conscious minds have no choice but to either accept their non-rational, undefinable nature for what it is, or to pretend that they do, in fact, fit into our rational framework, even though they don't.

In my experience, the latter is the course that most people take. After all, we can explain the entire surface of our worlds and everything that has ever happened in our lives by our rational understanding of things! Or can we?

I believe the truth is that everything on the surface of our worlds can only exist because of what's underneath. The underworld is the bedrock, the foundation of everything we know. And, frustratingly, we have little to no control over it. Just like with our actual physical planet, we can build all we like, but we're forever at the mercy of the shifting fault lines, which create shockwaves that can level even our most impressive structures in seconds. Entire cities can be washed away by a mudslide or tsunami. Sinkholes can open up and swallow buildings before we even realize what's happening. Most often, we're left at the site of the wreckage, confused and disappointed at the failure of our surface-level planning to prevent this disaster.

Frustrating and illogical though our fault lines and sub-surface landscapes may be, I think that we stand to gain enormously by seeking to understand and accept them as best we can. Which starts with admitting that this underworld exists. That our surface-level world is not at all lessened by what's underneath it (Yes, I'm talking to you, ego, settle down now!), but amplified instead. Sure, we can be hard-headed and insist that we can overpower our underworld through sheer force of will. We can ram our Titanic full speed into that iceberg, or build our major city right in the middle of a big fault line if we want, but at the end of the day, I believe there's a better option. That better option is to seek to understand and accept what our deeper layers look like.

Seeking to understand how we're blocking our energies is not about admitting fault. In fact, the very idea of fault is counter to celebration.

It's important to know that as you look deeper, you're probably not always going to like what you find. If you're anything like me, at times you'll be baffled, horrified, shocked, or disgusted at what's inside you. That's ok – that's par for the course of any significant self-reflection. In fact, I'd say that if you *don't* find yourself feeling distress at what you find, you're probably not digging deep enough. Remember that, by its very nature, our underworld does not conform in the slightest to the chosen values or beliefs of our surface mind.

If and when you find yourself feeling distressed at your discoveries, I would urge you to remember that even these deep truths do not define you. They are only one part of you, that you didn't even know existed until recently. *It is what you choose to do with your knowledge that defines you.* Responding with courage and compassion can allow us to mend our fault lines and create a whole self in which our parts are integrated harmoniously. Responding with rejection or judgement, on the other hand, hardens our deep parts and drives them even deeper, where they are even more disrupted and disharmonious.

When we live in harmony with our underworld, things align such that there are countless wellsprings of spiritual energy pouring forth throughout our surface world, fueling the building of greater and greater works. Every part of ourselves grows and flourishes when this energy is flowing. This is not likely to happen without a brave journey into our underworld to understand, accept, and then release the ways that we are blocking ourselves. None of us is without trauma, and I would go so far as to say that we all stand to benefit from taking the time to come to know ourselves on a deeper level.

The topic of journeying into our own personal underworlds is so vast that it deserves a book of its own, and there are many on the topic already. This journey is profoundly personal, and I'm certainly not qualified to comment on what you'll find there, or to guide you at all. Nobody is, really, except yourself. If you are interested in learning more on the topic, I would suggest that you read Bill Plotkin's Soulcraft, which puts the underworld journey into historical and cultural context, and gives an array of guiding principles and techniques that I have found helpful in my own journey.

Letting our ego take over

Another one of the ways that we mess up true celebration is when we make it about ourselves... Like this time!

It's not about you!

I am standing alone in the centre of the ring, in dead silence. Hundreds of eyes are trained on me, piercing through my skin, burrowing straight into my heart. Cold dread and panic fill my body. My hands are shaking, my body is drenched with sweat. It feels like I can barely remember my own name, much less perform the most difficult and complex skill I've ever had to perform. My knuckles turn white as they clench the juggling rings. The soldiers, with weapons in hand, shift on their feet, feeling the tension in the tent.

Back up a minute – how did I get myself into this mess? As you may have guessed, I had my damn ego to thank for this situation.

It's the summer of 2008. I'm travelling with the Festival Circus throughout England and Scotland. This is it, show #135, the final one of the season. It was our biggest challenge yet – to perform for the British military. The previous day, we'd been frisked, our caravans searched, as we pulled into the military base. 14-foot fences with razor wire, guards on duty 24/7 in tall towers and throughout the grounds, in full body armor, clutching assault rifles; all painted the scene. The following 24 hours were strangely eerie – erecting a circus tent and witnessing the set-up of a carnival midway in the deadly-serious atmosphere of a military base. We had a lightning storm to boot, an ill omen of what was to come...

The base was having its once-a-year celebration, and had hired our entire circus, along with a midway complete with bumper cars, ring-the-bell and other games. They paid to have our entire tent carpeted, for just one night. They built a wooden stage for us, and a set of tables, which were decorated, for the military officers to eat at while they watched our show. This was a far cry from our usual audience of casual festival-goers, families with children, and teens. Rather than being like a low-key community celebration, this felt more like an upper-class wedding. For military officers. With guards standing at the entrance to the tent, holding weapons. Needless to say, the pressure to perform was immense.

I had been working on a new trick all season. It's incredibly difficult, and took me the entire summer to learn. It's called a "6-ring pulldown". In it, you throw 6 juggling rings up into the air, and as they come down, one by one, you catch them and pull them down around your neck. The falling rings are separated by only about one tenth of a second...

That means that you need to fully catch the falling ring, without fumbling, and pull it down across your face onto your neck and clear your hand to allow the next ring to be pulled down, all within the space of a tenth of a second. Six times in a row without any error at all. And if you're even slightly inaccurate (we're talking a couple of degrees or milliseconds) on either your throw or your catch, it's pretty well impossible, and you risk scraping your nose or your ear clean off your head. Ok, maybe not, but it hurts like hell if you don't get it just right!

This being our final show, I wanted to make it special by putting in my new trick that I'd worked so hard on. I was excited about the show for several reasons – this circus tour had me working harder than I ever had in my life, for over 6 months straight, with barely a day or two off in that entire span of time. This show represented my last commitment before being free as a bird. Having joined the circus hot on the heels of finishing my university education, this show marked true freedom for the first time in my life, after nearly

20 consecutive years in educational institutions.

Our show began as normal, though our nerves were high. All of us were feeling the difference in context and the desire to end our tour on a high note. Act after act passed as I spent my time backstage practicing my new trick. I was feeling excited and nervous to get out there. My act was the final act of the show, an intense, fast-paced heavy metal juggling act featuring acrobatics, club, ball, and ring juggling. It was dynamic, high-energy, and exciting. Hence its place at the end of our show. With all my practice, I'm feeling confident as I bound out into the ring at a full run, executing a roundoff-backflip entrance (also a first for me). My act goes very well as a I land trick after trick. I can also feel the eyes of my comrades peeking from behind the curtains to see how the show ends.

Now, with the rest of the act completed, it's time for my final trick. I have a moment to survey the audience. It's composed of very upright-looking military officers in their full formal outfits, complete with medals of honour, and whatever other badges or commendations they had earned through their years of service. They are behaving as you'd expect any audience at a dinner show – they're eating and chatting with each other, with our show almost in the background. I realize that they might not know that this is the final trick of the show.

Well, after working so hard for all this time, I want to somehow communicate how significant this final trick is (anyone smell an ego here?). I reach back through my memory to some of the best circus acts I'd seen, and remember something that I had learned in my studies – when it comes to the most difficult part the act, circus artists sometimes play a little trick – they miss the first time **on purpose**, to build the tension and make it seem much more impressive when they succeed on the second try.

"I've got it!", I say in my mind: "I'll just miss on purpose the first time, and, it being the first time that I've dropped, they'll notice and pay close attention as I nail it on the second try!" Famous last words. I throw my rings up into the air – one, two, three, four, five, six. They're stacked perfectly – all my practice has paid off. One by one, I pull them down onto my head – one, two, three, four, five, and then I deliberately missed the last ring. It falls to the wooden floor with a loud crack. Heads turn.

"Great, I've got their attention now!", I think smugly in my head. My imagination is now running wild with the thunderous applause I expect to get when I smash the trick the second time around. In my head, I'm already lying on the beach somewhere, drink in hand, with fresh memories of my hard-earned accolades. "I did it – I finally made it to the end", I'm thinking. I throw the rings up into the air – one, two, three, four, five, six.

As you may have guessed, I didn't get off that easily...

"Oh shit!" I have only a moment to think before realizing how poorly I've thrown the rings. They're an absolute mess in the air, I can't possibly tell what order to catch them in, and some of them are going to land so far away that even if my arms had super-stretch powers, I still couldn't catch them. I do my best to fend off this barrage of falling props, catching one, two, and three, letting rings four, five, and six fall to the floor. They land noisily, and more heads turn. As I chase down my rings, which are rolling now in every direction, I feel flustered. Not confident at all. How could I have messed up so badly? No time to think about it now!

With a deep breath, I begin again. One, two, three, four, five, six. They're a little off, but I give it my best. I catch one, two, three, four, miss five, and catch six. Now I've failed the trick three times in a row. It's getting embarrassing. Looking out to the audience, I see their eyes on me, and I can feel what they're thinking – "Can he even do this?". And now **I'm** thinking – "**Can** I even do this?!"

See, when you're juggling, confidence is **extremely** important. Any doubt in your mind, any at all, will manifest in what you do. If you imagine yourself missing, you'll miss. Especially in the really difficult tricks. Standing there in front of the audience, I was feeling anything but confident.

So there I was, standing alone in the centre of the ring, in dead silence. My music has stopped. See, I was supposed to have finished my act, taken a bow, and gone back through the curtains. Filled with dread, I wonder what they hell I'm going to do if I can't get it. Just announce to the audience "Hey guys, sorry about that! Looks like I suck.... See you next *year!" You can't end a show that way!*

*Another deep breath. Try in vain to steady my panicking nerves. I throw the rings up into the air – one, two, three, four, five, six. I might be able to make it. I pull them down, one, two, three, notice something's off but keep going – four, five, and now.... I have a split second to make a decision. The sixth ring is pretty far away. I'm almost certainly not going to be able to catch it, and if I try, it'll throw me off balance. **But** – there's a small chance. A chance that, when the ring hits the wooden stage, it'll bounce back up. See, when you throw a juggling ring up and let it fall down to a hard floor, there's about a 50% chance that it'll clatter and wobble and fall over, and a 50% chance that it'll bounce perfectly back up into the air.*

With five rings around my neck, the audience on the edge of their seat, and less than a tenth of a second to decide, I choose to leave the ring. It hits the floor. Bouncing up, I snatch it out of the air and pull it down onto my head as the audience erupts from the sheer release of tension. The relief was greater than just about anything I had ever experienced in my life. Realizing what a fool I'd been, I vowed in that moment that I would never again miss a trick on purpose. That I would never again put my own gratification or indulgence above serving the audience.

My ego was entirely responsible for getting me into that mess. And I was damn lucky that it had a happy ending – I have no idea what I would have done if that ring hadn't bounced. You don't get unlimited tries in a situation like that. The audience didn't deserve the crappy ending that I *could easily have given them* because of my self-centredness. Over the following years, I came to appreciate the distinction between performing to make yourself look or feel good versus performing as an act of generosity to your audience.

Celebration has a similar distinction – if you're celebrating to stoke your ego, you might find yourself in a similar mess, looking like a fool and letting down the people you ought to be serving. If on the other hand you celebrate as an act of generosity and sharing, then even when things go wrong (as they often do), it's not so much a reflection on you. You're there to do your best, to *give yourself* to the thing you're celebrating, not to claim the riches or the status for yourself.

I still perform the six ring pulldown, complete with the story, feeling like a different person from the self-absorbed 20-year-old that got himself into that mess. I still make mistakes in front of audiences. As I mentioned, I'm not a great juggler, and my technique is far from perfect. But my audiences never seem to mind. I think that it's the act of celebration that they most connect with, much more than the success or failure of my silly tricks.

When I use juggling to celebrate the gifts that we are all born with as human beings, my audiences connect with the spirit behind it much more than the act itself. And the best thing is that it totally relieves me of the pressure of "getting it right". Which allows me to have fun and bring a light and positive energy with me rather than a dark and heavy one that makes people anxious to be around. Which brings me to the final point on how we get it wrong when it comes to celebration:

Evaluating & judging ourselves and others

I believe that the biggest enemy of celebration is evaluation and judgement. Nothing shuts us down quicker or more effectively than being judged. True celebration is based on the spirit of abundance, while judgement is based on the spirit of scarcity. To judge something as worthy or unworthy is based on the assumption that only certain things or people **can be** worthy. That is, it assumes that the title of "worthiness" is limited. That we only have five slots for worthiness, and now everything has to be judged and evaluated to determine if it gets the coveted prize of being deemed worthy.

But I ask – who the hell are we to think that we get to decide that? And furthermore, how absurd is it to think that anyone's sincere contribution is unworthy? That only certain art forms or expressions, or even people themselves, get to exist, and the rest should go away? Even if something doesn't appeal to us, that doesn't mean anything about their worthiness.

Even if you think of celebration in more literal terms – nothing kills the mood of a party quite like someone going around complaining about the dip, how the music sucks, and that this isn't nearly as good as that party they went to last week. Imagine then the further audacity of throwing the food out the window, interrupting the concert, and taking over the microphone to tell everyone how they're not doing it right. Who the hell wants to party in a context like that? That's what judgement does to celebration. It says that if the food isn't good enough, it's going out the window. And that if the band isn't good enough, the gong will sound and they'll be kicked out. And that if the art isn't good enough, it's getting torn down from the walls.

Judgment tells us that there's only one shot and that we have to get it right. That it's a terrible crime when we don't. It totally kills the mood, and puts us on edge. It then sparks our inner critic that stifles everything from the inside. And that's no damn way to live your life! I believe the truth is that you don't only get one shot – every day, every moment, is a new chance to celebrate. That no one (including you!) is qualified to judge the merit of your deeds. The simple fact that you can do what you do is a miracle, a gift from the divine, and we have no right to sully it with our petty judgements. It is that spirit of abundance and joy that gives celebration its power to transform, to ignite, to bring light to the world around us.

How to come back

We're all guilty of being hijacked by our egos, of living in disharmony with ourselves, and of judging ourselves and others. It's ok – it arises from the same miraculous capacity for creating and appreciating beauty. So rather than blaming ourselves for blaming ourselves, let's celebrate that too! Celebrate that we have the ability to distinguish what's favourable from what's unfavourable. What we like from what we don't like. As long as we don't let those distinctions prevent us (or others) from creating what we feel inspired to create, there's nothing wrong with them! Celebrate that we can know what we like and what we don't like. Celebrate that we've developed an understanding of the "right" and "wrong" ways of doing things (just don't get too attached to those labels - you know they're bunk, right?). Can you imagine what life would be like if we *didn't* have that capacity? We'd literally have to reinvent the wheel every time we made a new car, bicycle, or unicycle!

Let's just also remember to let our ideas of "right" and "wrong" go when they don't serve us. That there are many many many "right" ways for anything, more than our individual minds could ever conceive of. And that the "wrong" ways of doing things often pave the way for the "right" ways. Accept that we may not even have the wisdom to be able to separate the two! All of this is worth celebrating because it's all part of the miraculous package of being human. Our incredible capacity to have all kinds of thoughts, to be in conflict with ourselves, to represent more than one viewpoint, is stupendous. It really truly is a miracle, which is allowed to unfold when we can teach ourselves to see it that way.

Coming back to celebration begins with realizing that even our capacity for *not* celebrating is worth celebrating. It's remembering that **joy is in the ears that hear it.** Are *you* listening?

Conclusion

You shouldn't need a special invitation to be able to stand up and celebrate. The simple fact that you **can** should be enough. But, in case it's not, here's your special invitation:

Stand up! Celebrate!

Have you got two functional arms?

Great! Use them!

Get out a hammer and pound in some nails!

Learn to juggle!

Give a really great back massage to someone!

Got legs? Great!

Go for a run! Climb some stairs!

Learn how to do a backflip!

Got a mind? Incredible!

Use it to solve puzzles!

Learn a new language!

Learn something new from someone who thinks very differently than you.

Why?

Because you can, dammit!

What if you were trapped in a cage for a week and couldn't use your arms or legs, or have access to the internet or another person? What's the first thing you'd want to do when you got out? Use your body, I bet! Stretch out, jump for joy, have a conversation with *anyone*! Well, what's stopping you from doing that now? I think you're probably still trapped in that cage of your mind, constrained by bars of your own creation. Well, here's your invitation to leave that behind, to enter a world where there's no evaluation, there's just the joy of doing the things that matter to you.

Here we are at the end, and yet find ourselves back at the beginning. Such is the cyclical nature of life and learning. You can see how this final rule folds back into the first one – believe it's possible. I'm bringing you back there because chances are you need a reminder at this point. We all do!

In case it would be helpful, I'll also give you permission to have your interests be wacky and wild and crazy (as long as they don't mess with other people's liberty to do the same). Surround yourself with people who are also weird and wacky, and have weird wacky parties together! Your interests don't have to be the same as mine. And they don't have to go anywhere "productive" either.

Simply having an interest, I believe, is worth celebrating. And celebrating is as simple as pursuing that interest wherever it takes you.

And don't tell me that you don't have interests – I don't believe that for a second. I believe that you may *feel* that way, but if you do, it's only because you *had* an interest, and then dismissed it. Why did you do it? I don't know… maybe you did it to protect yourself from failure, or from mockery from the world around you. Maybe you did it because you judged your own interest as being trivial. Maybe it was too expensive or too dangerous or too difficult.

But you've got to understand that you're paying a big cost when you do this. Every time you shut down an idea or an interest, you're secretly signalling to all of the other ideas or interests waiting on the outskirts of your mind that they might get cut next. Suddenly they all flock in the other direction, and you're left vacant, without anything compelling to do with yourself. Then you have no choice but to look to the world outside you to entertain you, to fill the void where your interests should live and flourish. If you shut down too many of your own ideas, you've ripped up your whole garden and soon you'll find yourself peeking into all your neighbours' yards, both envious and judgemental, but never satisfied.

Remember that joy is in the ears that hear it – are you listening? Really, truly listening? Because it's out there, and will never cease to be. Even if you have a million terrible experiences in your life. As long as your ears are prepared to hear it, there is joy all around us.

I acknowledge that there are also some pretty bad, twisted things in our world. But none of that means that there's no beauty. It just means that there's also ugliness. I'm not suggesting that our world is all rosy and beautiful all the time.

What I think is most incredible is that we can carry on *despite all that ugliness*. That, as black as things may get, we still have the capacity for action, for meaning and for celebration. That, even if something terrible happens to us, we can still choose to celebrate. No, it's not easy, but why should it be? And furthermore, who cares if it's easy?

As I related earlier, I've been through some really rough times. And, though I wouldn't ever claim to understand somebody else's experiences of suffering, I believe that, regardless of the depths of our suffering, we always retain the ability to choose what we do with it. And if you can't bring yourself to believe privileged Andrew on this one - read Viktor Frankl.

To inject a bit of perspective here, I want to reference a great comedian of our time – Louis CK. I've always appreciated Louis' ability to not get swept up in our bizarre culture of entitlement.

*Life is short. Life is very short. I like life... I feel like, even if it ends up being short, I got lucky to have it. 'Cause life is an amazing gift when you think about what you get with a basic life. Not even a particularly lucky life. Or a healthy life. If you **have** a life, it's amazing... Here's your boilerplate deal with life. This is basic cable, what you get, when you get life. You get to be on **earth**. First of all, **oh my GOD** what a location! This is Earth, and for trillions of miles in every direction, it f***ing sucks SO BAD, it's so sh*tty that your eyes bolt out of your head 'cause it sucks so bad. You get to be on earth and look at sh*t. As long as you're not blind, or whatever... You get to be here, you get to eat **food**. You get to put **bacon** in your mouth. I mean, when you have bacon in your mouth, it doesn't matter who's president, or anything! Everytime I'm eating bacon, I think 'I could die right now,' and **I mean it**! That's how good life is.*

When we celebrate, our capacities are increased tremendously. When we add energy into the world, it responds in kind. The gift of service is twofold – you help increase the capacity of those around you while also increasing your own. So get out there and do your thing - no one else can do it for you!

I'd like to share with you a great quote that is often misattributed to Nelson Mandela. The actual author is Marianne Williamson:

Our deepest fear is not that we are inadequate. Our deepest fear is that we are powerful beyond measure. It is our light, not our darkness that most frightens us. We ask ourselves, Who am I to be brilliant, gorgeous, talented, and fabulous? Actually, who are you not to be? You are a child of God. Your playing small does not serve the world. There is nothing enlightened about shrinking so that other people will not feel insecure around you. We are all meant to shine, as children do. We were born to make manifest the glory of God that is within us. It is not just in some of us; it is in everyone and as we let our own light shine, we unconsciously give others permission to do the same. As we are liberated from our own fear, our presence automatically liberates others.

Make no mistake – sharing our gifts is painful. Being sincerely present, and following the wisdom of juggling will lead to pain. As I'm sure some famous person once said: "Haters gonna hate." That's the cost of entry in this game of life - you're going to have to deal with criticism, judgment, obfuscation, restriction, even downright opposition. But really, what the hell else are you going to do? Live your life deliberately switched off because it's sometimes less painful? Nonsense! You'll still have problems, they'll just be about things you don't care about rather than things you do!

One last point on the subject of the pain related to sharing your gifts. When you lean into the challenge of it, with sincerity and presence, it can sometimes feel unbearable. When people around you don't take you seriously, when it feels like you're butting your head against the wall, when you're failing left and right, you mustn't lose heart. It can, and will, feel like there's no point during these hard times. But even if you're not making any measurable external progress, you are benefiting nonetheless. Your pain will make you stronger. The more adversity you face, the more that you'll be able to handle in the future.

If your path were straight and easy, it wouldn't mean all that much. People that are born rich don't generally appreciate what they've got. It is precisely because you have to pay so dearly for the gift that you bring to the world that it is worth so much. Just don't let the pain along the way harden your heart and forget the joy that's possible in celebration. Remember your juggling wisdom and carry it with you always!

Thank you for taking the time to read my words. I am humbled and grateful for the chance to share! If you'd like to discuss any of the ideas I touched on, I'd love to learn from you. If you feel moved enough to share your thoughts, I will commit to taking the time to read them!

Afterword

What's that? It's not finished yet? Ah, yes! I promised I'd share the ending of our Prologue story before we're done. Where were we again? Oh yeah, preparing to juggle "razor-sharp" knives 200 feet up in the air.

> As I mentioned, I had to wear this awkward chest-strapped phone carrier, which looked (and felt) like some horrible alien arm bursting forth from my chest and reaching right into my face. It completely threw off my balance, and occupied the whole space in which I would normally have juggled. To boot, the slackline I was standing on was WAY tighter than I was used to.
>
> To give some context, I have the skills and confidence to walk on a tightwire, which doesn't move at all, or on a stretchy, swaying slackline. They require vastly different balancing techniques. But this felt like some strange hybrid of the two - it moved much more than a tightwire (in fact, it was vibrating like a firing machine gun in the intense wind), but not enough for me to use the typical hip-swaying slackline balance technique. So neither skill set applied, and I was completely out of my element with an antsy audience, high winds, high altitude, and some dorky thing attached to my chest.
>
> To give a window into my thinking at the time, I was pretty well pooping my pants here. I mean, I've done ridiculous stuff in my time, but this was WAY outside my normal "danger"

performances. My anxiety level was ultra-high. Luckily, by this point in my career, I knew how to deliver results despite the anxiety. It no longer had the power to faze me the way it once did.

As for the skills, I knew enough to know that there was a very significant possibility of screwing up. And I was very close to the edge of the building - a small stumble could very well launch me over the side, and down 200 feet to my death. Or if I had a collision of the knives in the air, not only would I be in danger, so would the audience, and so would the passersby on the sidewalk way down below.

With the pressure on, and no time to lose, you may be able to guess what I did next. I used my Juggling Wisdom. I believed that it was possible. In the face of true uncertainty, I chose to tell the story of how I would get out of this. And by god, I committed to it! There was really no room at all to doubt myself at this point.

I made sure to tell a realistic story of what I was going to do - I would juggle for the tiniest amount of time I could and stop immediately. I "dropped the ball" (not actually dropping the knives, but certainly dropping the expectations of myself and the audience that it was going to be some great big thing). I threw each of the three knives exactly once, caught them, and immediately jumped off the slackline onto the solid ground of the rooftop, and moved to step three - I celebrated.

And, ooh boy, did I ever celebrate! I cheered so loudly that I drowned out the crowd, who were uncertain how to react to the eye-blinkingly-short juggling act. I declared that it was a victory, and I did so with such energy and enthusiasm that the audience had no choice but to go along with it.

I shouted at the top of my lungs and let the energy pour through every part of my body. I then joked "Yeah! it was short. But hey, it's better than any of you could do!" The audience exploded in laughter and relief. The release of tension was enough to make it hilarious to the crowd.

And who could argue? I did, in fact, juggle the knives on the slackline, despite the many (and very good) reasons why it should have been impossible, and to boot, I didn't die, and even ended with a joke! What more could an audience want?

The truth is, anxiety never goes away. It's one of the many colours of the tapestry of life. Railing against it never moves us forward. The only thing that does is to calmly defy it. To take your story back and declare that you are too strong to let your anxiety make your choices for you. Remember - your goal is not to get rid of the anxiety, your goal is to put it firmly into the category of "overcomeable obstacles".

There is nothing wrong with you for having anxiety. If getting on the bus, or paying for your groceries, or delivering a presentation to your class/coworkers, or even tying your shoe gives you anxiety, that doesn't mean a damn thing about who you are or your value as a human. Arguing with yourself about whether you should or shouldn't be anxious about something is not only a waste of time, it's bound to end with you angry at yourself. And you don't deserve that!

One last note - a decade and a half into my journey, I still have anxiety in a variety of mundane situations. I always feel overwhelmed when preparing for any performance or professional speaking work. Every single time. I get nervous talking to people, and most often prefer to stay home. I still hate checking out and bagging my groceries. But every time I find myself in one of those situations, I carry with me the knowledge of all of my victories, and all of my capabilities. I recognize the anxiety for what it is - a feeling that will pass, that has no power at all to determine my limits. If I ever choose to avoid the anxiety and hide in something easy, I at least know that I don't *have to*. I can *choose* to take the easy way, and still know that I'm capable of taking the hard way.

Appendix

Intro to juggling

     Welcome to the Juggling Section of the book! After all that talk, you're probably itching to get your hands dirty, so to speak! For this section, you're going to need some balls. Don't worry, you don't actually need proper juggling balls for this – they would make it a bit easier, but we're certainly not going to skip this if you haven't got any.
     You can use just about any grabbable object you've got on hand for this. Some examples would be handheld fruit (apples and oranges – yes. Banana or watermelon – probably a lot trickier), a tennis ball, dog ball, or road hockey ball, heck, even a shoe will work in a pinch! But let's say you're stranded on a desert island without any of the above objects... Don't you worry! Your dear pal Andrew has you covered – The final 3 pages of the book are left blank and intended to be ripped out and crumpled up to use as juggling balls!

(Unless you've got the digital version, in which case, you can crumple up the imaginary digital page. And yes, it *does work* - your brain would look almost exactly the same if it were scanned juggling real or imagined objects!)

So, grab your nearest juggling-appropriate object, and let's get started!

Exercise One: The One-Ball Box

Step One – Side-to-side throws

    There are many different types of throws in the world of juggling. We're going to start with a straight throw. This is where the ball travels directly in a straight line from one hand to the next. You can even start out with a handoff if the throw is too tricky, and work your way up to a throw.

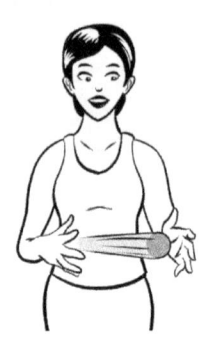

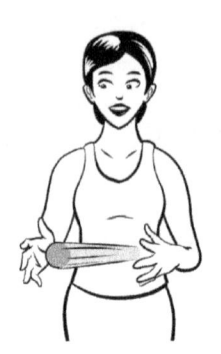

...Pretty easy, right? When you're comfortable, move on to...

Step Two – Vertical throws
    Reach one hand up over the other, and throw the ball straight up to the waiting hand. Close your hand at the exact moment the ball reaches it. Keeping your top hand directly over your bottom hand, release the ball and let it fall back down into your bottom hand. Once you've got it on the one side, switch your top and bottom hands.

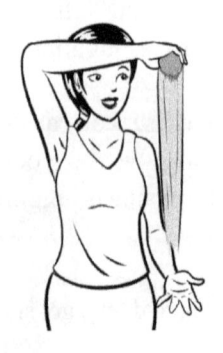

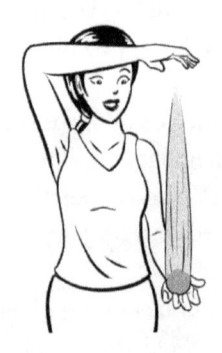

Switch!

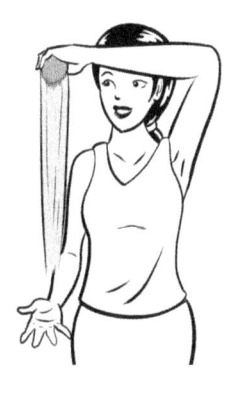

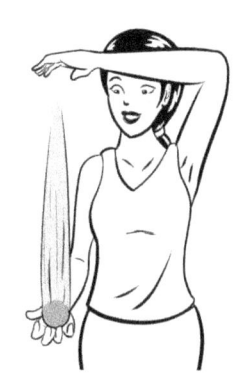

Alright! Now you're ready for your first trick – it's called "Anti-gravity". Throw the ball up as normal. Keeping the ball in your top hand, switch your hand positions, and throw up to your new top hand. Throw up again, and switch. Throw up, switch. That's right, folks – the secret to juggling… is throwing up!

Anti-gravity

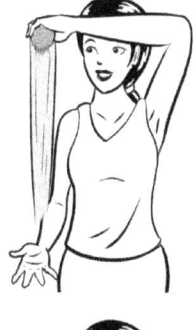

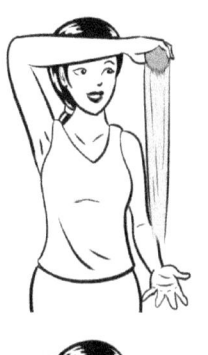

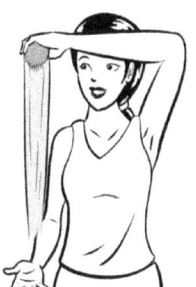

Switch!

Switch!

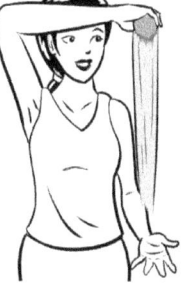

When you get the motion smooth, it looks like the ball is falling in reverse. Hence the name, Anti-gravity! You can also try the trick backwards – drop and switch, drop and switch. This one's called "Reverse Anti-gravity". Or, you know, just regular gravity.

Reverse Anti-Gravity

Switch!

Switch!

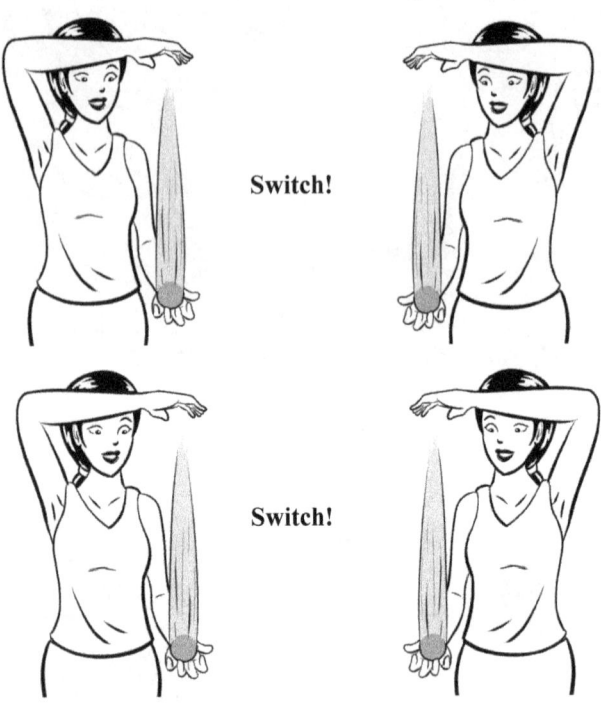

Step Three – The One-Ball Box
We're finally here! Ready at last to put all the pieces together for your first multi-part juggling trick! It's called the One-Ball Box, because you're making a box shape in the air, using only one ball.

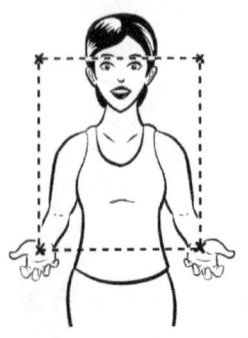

Four corners of the box

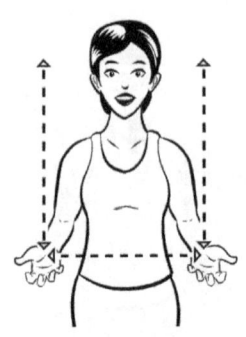

Path that the ball takes

Ready? Go!

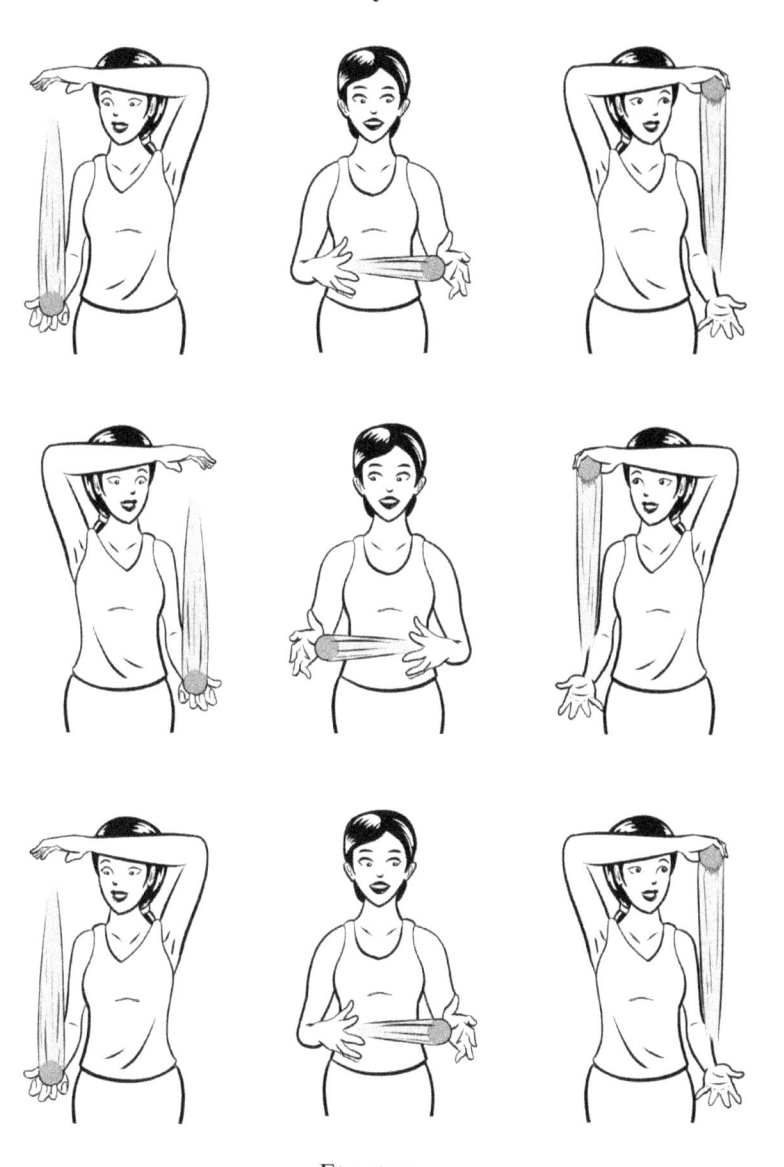

Et cetera...

If you get lost, just repeat the following narration in your head: Up, down, across. Up, down, across. When you speed the pattern up, it makes the shape of a box with no lid.

Congratulations! You can now juggle!

Exercise Two: The Figure Eight

The next one-ball trick I teach is a bit more complex than the linear pattern we've just gone through. We'll start out the same way, but eventually end with your hands executing an impressive series of orbits around the ball as it travels through the air. Don't worry - it's pretty easy to follow when I break it down.

Step One - One-handed vertical throws

This one begins with a vertical throw that starts and ends in the same hand, while your other hand does nothing. Visualize the apex of the throw - it's the same point that your other hand would catch the ball in the previous trick. Practice keeping the apex at a consistent height. In juggling, your aim is consistency and accuracy. Practice the vertical throw one hand at a time until both sides feel comfortable. Note that the ball remains centred with the body on this throw.

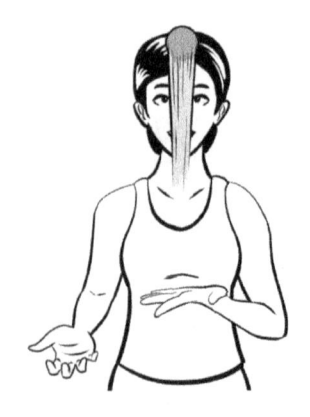

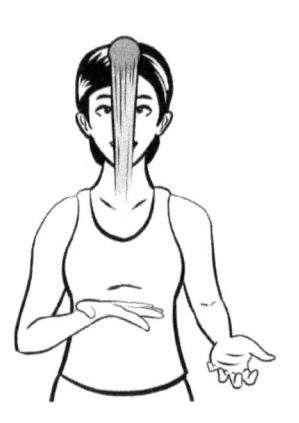

Step Two - Throw, cross-over, catch

Now it's time for that lazy arm to get involved by executing a completely irrelevant action while your throwing arm does exactly the same thing. While the ball is on its journey upward, you will pass your arm beneath the ball and across your body to the opposite side. Leave it there as the ball falls back into your throwing hand. You will end with one arm in neutral position and the opposite arm across your body. Throw again and return your crossed arm to neutral while the ball is airborne. Once you get the hang of it, practice the throw-cross-catch action on the other side. Don't worry - neither part of this is difficult, it just feels like a bit of a brain twister until you've done it a few times, and then you won't even have to think about it!

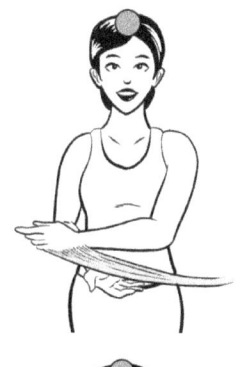

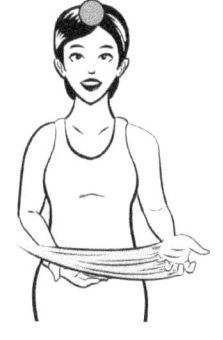

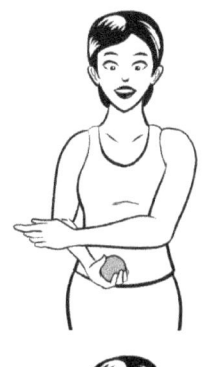

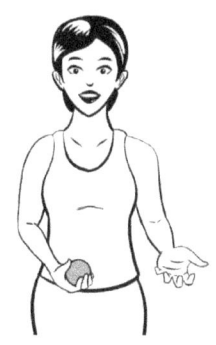

Switch!

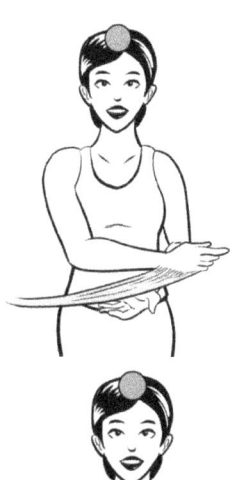

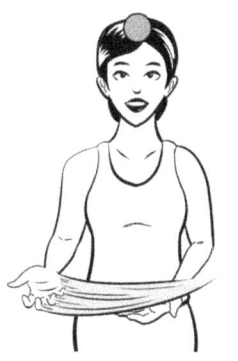

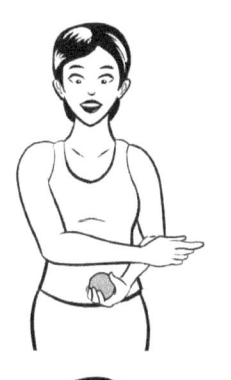

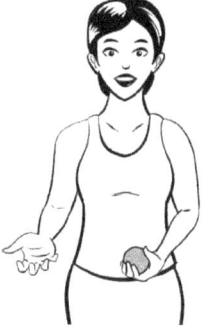

Step Three - Throw, orbit, catch
    Once you can perform step two without thinking or difficulty, you're ready to start the orbit. All you have to do is the same pass-under-the-ball motion, but this time, instead of staying put there, your hand will return to neutral by passing above the ball while it's in the air in a circular motion.

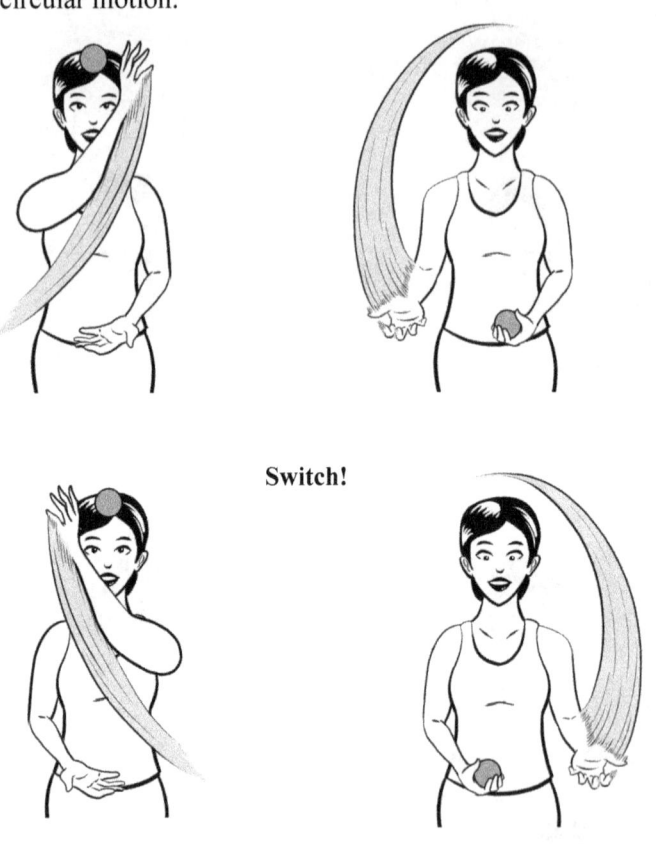

Switch!

Incredible! You're so good at this! Only one step to go!

Step Four - Throw, orbit, catch *with orbiting hand*
    Next, you're going to make sure that you do your orbit quickly enough that your orbiting hand returns to neutral **before the ball lands.** When your orbits are fast and consistent enough for this, **you can now catch the ball with your orbiting hand.**

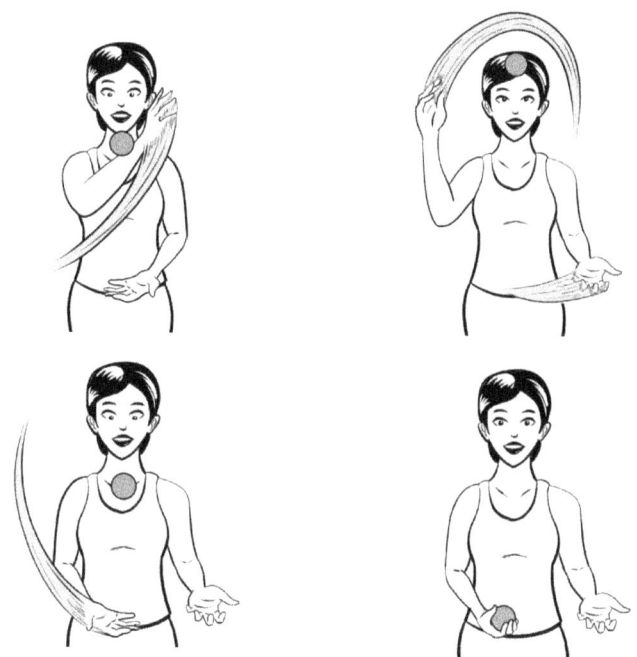

Notice which hand catches here.

Now the ball is in your other hand, ready to repeat the cycle.

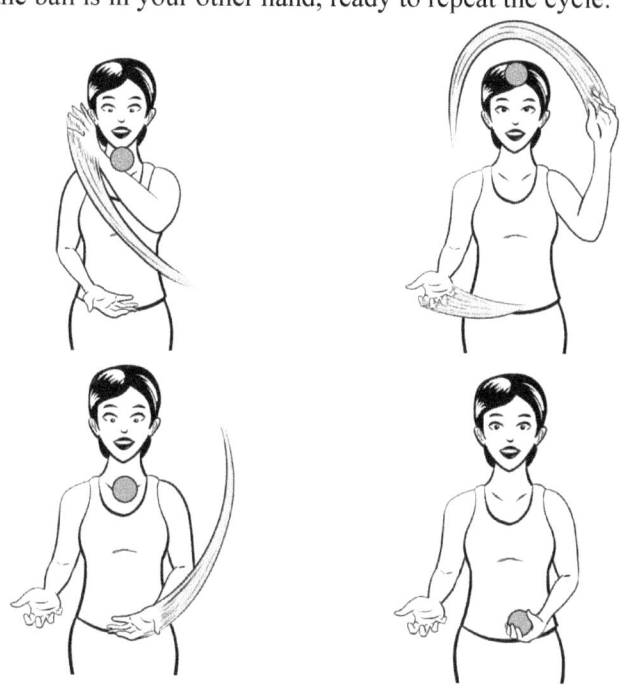

Hooray! You did it!

At this point, you may or may not notice that your pattern probably looks a bit different from the one pictured here. That's great! In fact, I think that it's a greater sign of success than if you were able to replicate this pattern exactly. Why? Because when you deviate from the source material, it shows that you've added your own flavour. Your brain is different from mine, so why *should* your pattern look the same as mine?

When I teach this pattern in my juggling workshops, I usually take a moment to explain the different ways that the pattern could look - your throws *could* look like a figure-8, swooping from left to right and back. Or they could be straight up and down in the center (as illustrated in this book). Your arms may be making great big swooping motions or very small and tight orbits. A small percentage of people can't help but catch the ball in the middle of the orbit rather than coming all the way around with their hands. Not sure why - their brains seem to be wired to work that way.

The great news is: it's all correct! I believe very strongly that there is *no right/wrong way to juggle*, just like there's no right/wrong way to live life. It's up to you to make it your own, and no one on this planet has the right to tell you that you're doing it wrong... Unless you're getting all up in my biz, in which case, please stop! But this isn't a book about ethics, it's a book about believing that your way is just as valid (and worth celebrating!) as any other.

You may be thinking "But Andrew, if I drop the ball all the time and never catch it, *that's* not juggling! How can you say that dropping the ball every time isn't wrong?"

Enter bounce juggling. There is, in fact, an entire school of juggling where you deliberately drop the ball. Every single time. There are specially designed juggling balls that retain over 90% of the height on each bounce. Do a quick search of bounce juggling, I promise your mind will be blown by what's out there. It's a perfect example of a way to turn "mistakes" into something spectacular!

...What's that? You want more?! Well, buckle up my friend - it's time to double up!

Two-ball Juggling Patterns

Well, since I haven't scared you off yet, let's keep going! Next, we're going to take a look at the building blocks you've already learned, and combine them in new ways.

Exercise 3: The Two-Ball Box

Step One - Back & forth

We're going to start with only one ball, doing the same side-to-side throw as with the one-ball box. Only this time, you're going to do exactly two throws, back and forth, as quickly as you can.

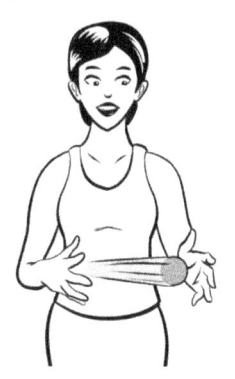

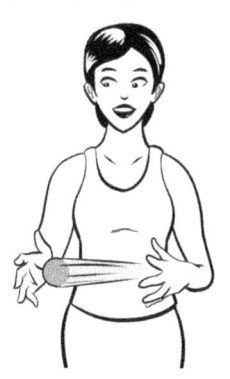

In this step, it's important to do only two throws and stop. You're building a pattern that will help considerably for the next step, but it'll only help if it's exactly two throws.

Step Two - The Box

Take the second ball, and throw it straight up in the air. While it's in the air, pass the original ball back and forth underneath. At first, it won't feel like you have enough attention to spare for these two separate actions at the same time.

The good news is that it's actually only the *illusion* of two actions at once. In fact, as soon as the first (vertical) ball leaves your hand, you can almost forget about it completely, and shift your attention to the second (horizontal) ball. There is actually plenty of time for both actions, as long as you start them at the right time!

I like to suggest that, immediately after the first ball has left your hands, you start the second ball back and forth between hands. With a bit of practice, you'll probably notice that it becomes nearly effortless and you don't even have to think about it! Thanks, brain!

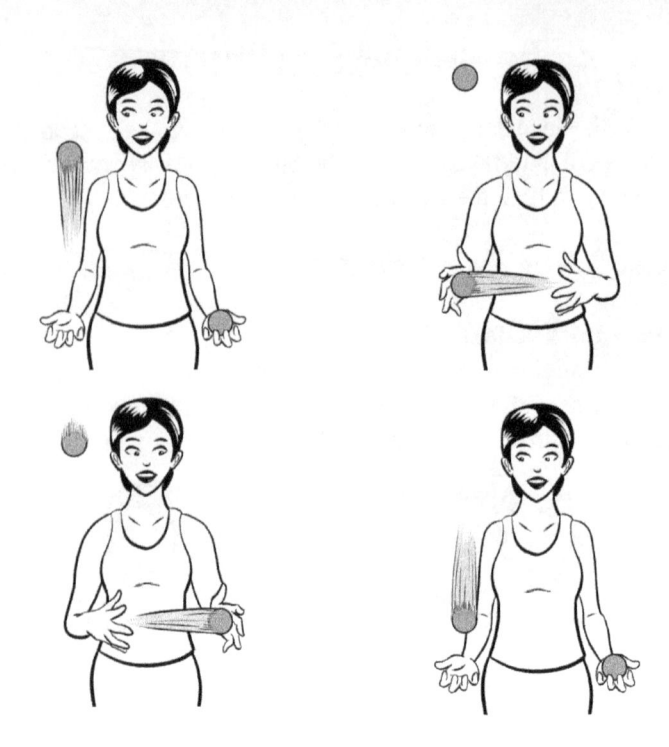

Once you feel confident in the process, you can switch sides.

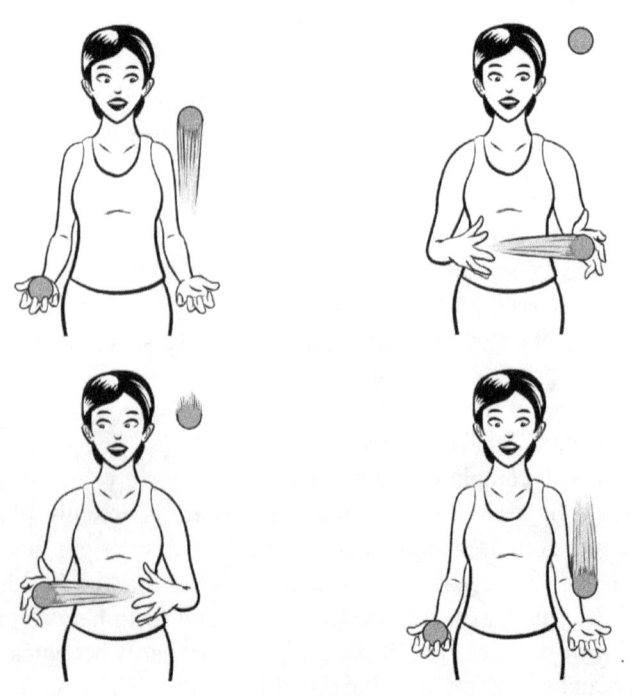

When you can perform the pattern well and quickly on each side, you'll see just how satisfying it is. It looks quite impressive too! If I was there in person, I'd give you a pat on the back. Since I'm not, you'll have to do it for me!

Exercise 4: The Two-Ball Shower

Very similar to the two-ball box, the next trick is the stereotypical juggling pattern that most people will do automatically if given two juggling balls. It's what those clowns in kids books are always doing - somehow creating an impossible circle of the balls in the air. In reality, it's not quite a circle. More like a semi-circle, or semi-oval.

The big difference between the shower and the box is that the vertical throw makes a "rainbow" shape as it passes from one hand to the other (rather than coming back to the hand that launched it). The balls end up in opposite hands rather than in the same hands.

Step One - The Rainbow

Practice with one ball, throwing it to the height of your head, from one hand to the other. Try not to exaggerate the rainbow shape though - it'll force your hands pretty wide if you do this, which makes the next step more difficult.

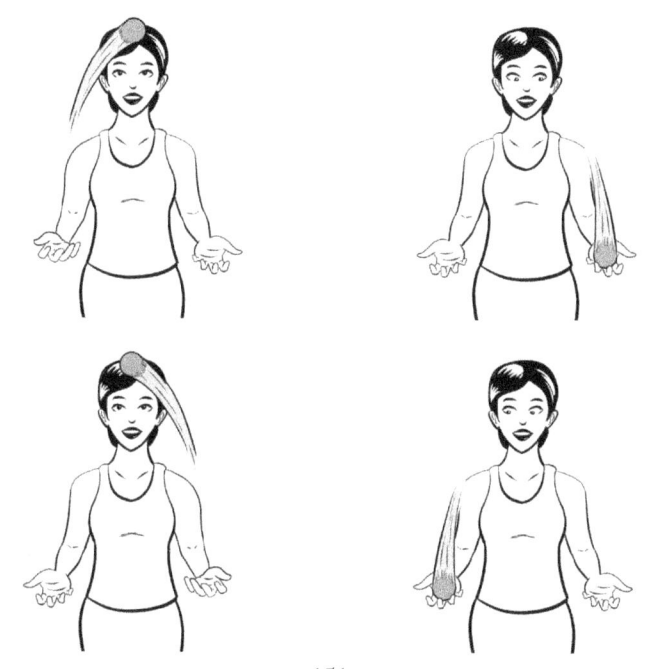

Step Two - The Shower

    This time, hold one ball in each hand. Throw the first ball in the arc you've just practiced. While it's in the air, your catching hand needs to be cleared - do this by passing the ball in it directly over to the other side.

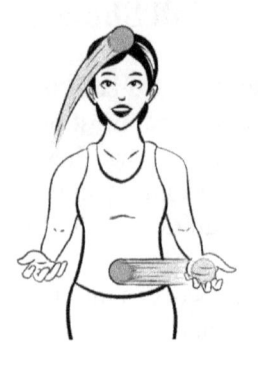

Step Three - Repeat!

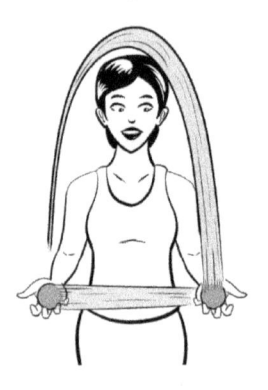

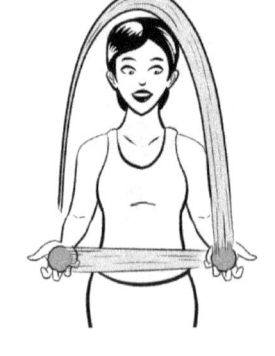

Step Four - Reverse!

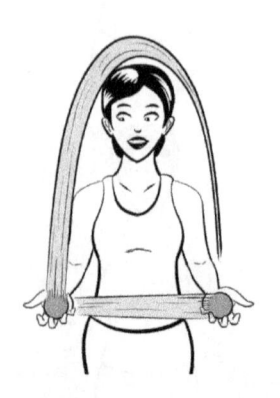

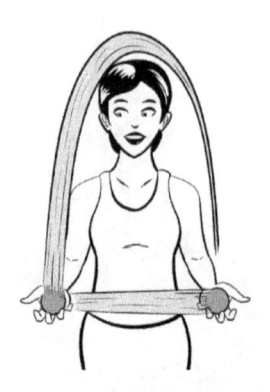

Incredible! If I were there, I'd give you a high five. I'm not, so you'll have to put the balls down for a moment and give yourself a high five!

Exercise 5: Your Turn!

Alright, you've just spent a bunch of time listening to *my* advice and doing all the things *I've* said.

...You *did* do them, right?

Well, now it's your turn! You have enough of the building blocks - I certify that you are ready to strike out on your own, to make a new pattern, and to tell *me* what to do! Get creative! Make me work for it!

No, really - I invite you to come up with a new pattern and teach me. I love learning new things. Hell, it doesn't even have to be a juggling pattern, I'd just love to hear from you! I promise that I'll take the time to respond if you do. Send me a video, a picture, even some text, and I'll give your ideas some space in my brain, and let you know what I think!

Now, I'm an old-fashioned guy, so you can really only reach me through telegram or carrier pigeon... Just kidding! Well, mostly. For real though, I'm not on social media, so don't bother looking. But I do promise I'll get back to you if you send me an email at:

JugglingAndrew@gmail.com

Looking forward to hearing from you!

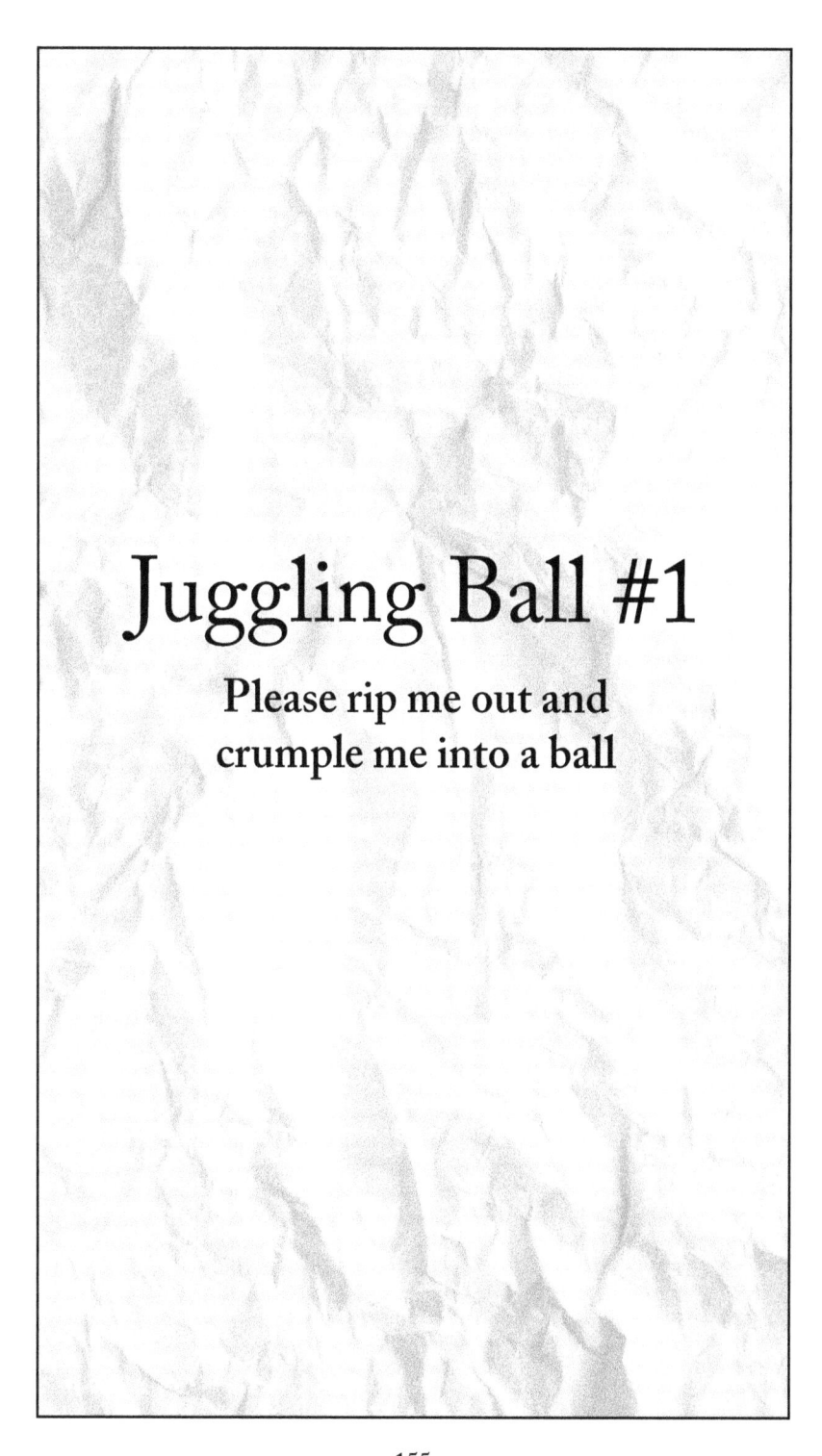

Juggling Ball #1

Please rip me out and crumple me into a ball

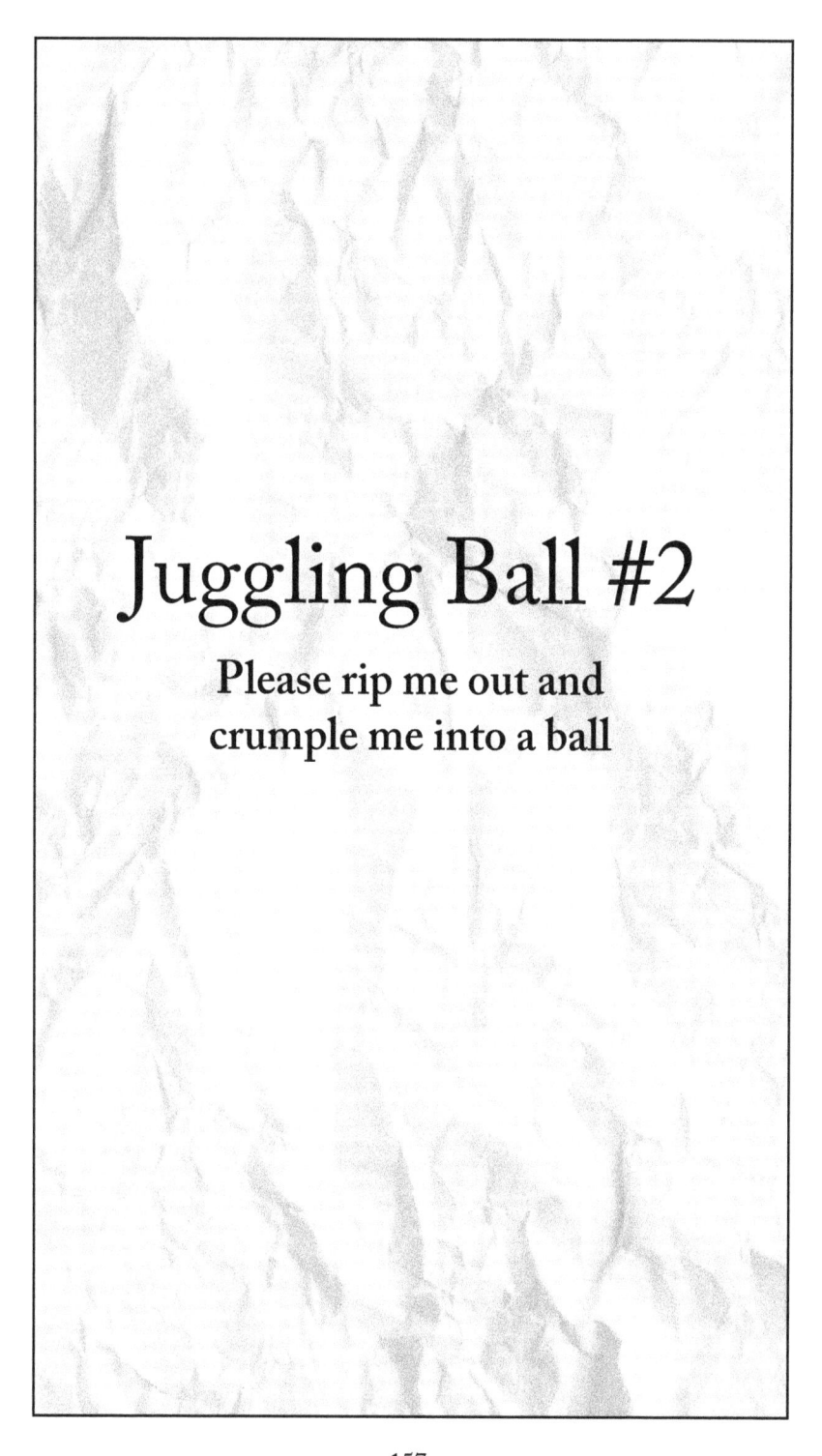

Juggling Ball #2

Please rip me out and crumple me into a ball

Juggling Ball #3

Please rip me out and crumple me into a ball

The Paper Game
Use me for this. And good luck.

Attempt #1

The Paper Game
Use me for this. And good luck.

Attempt #2

The Paper Game

Use me for this. And good luck.

Attempt #3

CPSIA information can be obtained
at www.ICGtesting.com
Printed in the USA
BVHW080725031221
622949BV00002B/20